Plastic and Hand Surgery
in Clinical Practice

Plastic and Hand Surgery in Clinical Practice
Classifications and Definitions

Mary O'Brien, MPhil, FRCS (Plast)

*Consultant Plastic and Hand Surgeon,
Pulvertaft Hand Centre, Derby, UK*

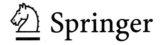 Springer

Mary O'Brien, MPhil, FRCS (Plast)
Consultant Plastic and Hand Surgeon
Pulvertaft Hand Centre
Derby
UK

ISBN 978-1-84800-262-3   e-ISBN 978-1-84800-263-0
DOI: 10.1007/978-1-84800-263-0

British Library Cataloguing in Publication Data

Library of Congress Control Number: 2008936262

© Springer-Verlag London Limited 2009
Apart from any fair dealing for the purposes of research or private study, or criticism
or review, as permitted under the Copyright, Designs and Patents Act 1988,
this publication may only be reproduced, stored or transmitted, in any form or by
any means, with the prior permission in writing of the publishers, or in the case
of reprographic reproduction in accordance with the terms of licences issued by the
Copyright Licensing Agency. Enquiries concerning reproduction outside those terms
should be sent to the publishers.
The use of registered names, trademarks, etc. in this publication does not imply, even in
the absence of a specific statement, that such names are exempt from the relevant laws
and regulations and therefore free for general use.
Product liability: The publisher can give no guarantee for information about drug
dosage and application thereof contained in this book. In every individual case the
respective user must check its accuracy by consulting other pharmaceutical literature.

Printed on acid-free paper

springer.com

To my parents in whose footsteps I aspire to follow
To my husband whose footsteps I walk alongside
To my children whose footsteps I chase

Preface

THE PLASTIC SURGEON'S CREED
Millard DR, Jr

"Know the ideal beautiful normal. Diagnose what is present; what is diseased, destroyed, displaced or distorted; and what is in excess. Then, guided by the normal in your mind's eye, use what you have to make what you want- and when possible go for even better than what would have been."

THE PRINCIPLES OF PLASTIC SURGERY
Gillies HD, Millard DR, Jr: The Principles and Art of Plastic Surgery. 1st Ed Boston. Little, Brown & Co 1957.

"Plastic surgery is a constant battle between blood supply and beauty.
Observation is the basis of surgical diagnosis.
Diagnose before you treat.
Make a plan and a pattern for this plan.
Make a record- sketches and photographs.
The lifeboat another flap or skin graft.
A good style will get you through- dexterity and gentleness.
Replace what is normal in normal position and retain it there.
Treat the primary defect first - borrow from Peter to pay Paul only when Peter can afford it.
Losses must be replaced in kind.
Do something positive- start with a landmark or two pieces that definitely fit.
Never throw anything away- a preserved piece may be used later.
Never let routine methods be your master.
Consult other specialists.
Speed in surgery consists of not doing the same thing twice.

The aftercare is as important as the planning.

Never do today what can honourably be put off till tomorrow- when in doubt, don't.

Time, although the plastic surgeon's most trenchant critic, is also his greatest ally."

Acknowledgements

I would like to express sincere thanks to Mr Keith Allison FRCS (Plast) and Mr Darren Chester FRCS (Plast) for their contributions in proof reading the manuscript.

I am particularly grateful to the many trainers both medical and those in professions allied to medicine for their teaching, encouragement, and support.

I also gratefully acknowledge the assistance and immense resources made available to me by the excellent library staff at University Hospitals Coventry & Warwickshire NHS Trust.

Without the helpful assistance of the team at Springer- Verlag, this book would not have been published.

Without the support of my family, this book would never have been written. Thank you.

Contents

Chapter 1
Fundamentals of Plastic Surgery

Plastic Surgery
    Greek derivation–"Plastikos" = "To mould"

1.1   A "SURGICAL SIEVE"
A useful filter to obtain a pathological diagnosis

Congenital
or
Acquired – Trauma
          – Tumour
          – Infective
          – Inflammatory
          – Metabolic
          – Endocrine
          – Iatrogenic

1.2   THE "RECONSTRUCTIVE LADDER" (FIGURE 1.1)
An evaluation of increasingly complex techniques to achieve
wound closure:

Free tissue transfer (complex)
Regional flap
Local flap
Skin graft (split thickness or full thickness, meshed or unmeshed,
skin substitutes)
Direct closure
Secondary intention healing (simple or vacuum therapy)

1

Mary O'Brien, *Plastic and Hand Surgery in Clinical Practice*,
DOI: 10.1007/978-1-84800-263-0_1,
© Springer-Verlag London Limited 2009

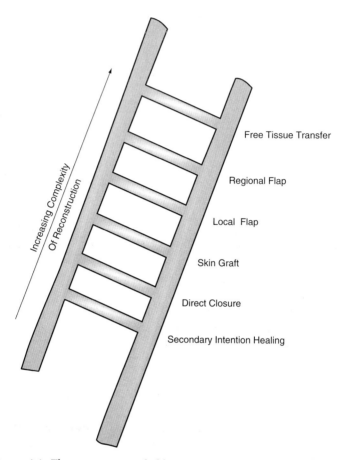

Free Tissue Transfer

Regional Flap

Local Flap

Skin Graft

Direct Closure

Secondary Intention Healing

Increasing Complexity Of Reconstruction

FIGURE 1.1. The reconstructive ladder.

1.3 FRAMEWORK FOR ANSWERING A QUESTION
Incidence
Aetiology/age
Sex distribution
Geographical
Symptoms and signs
Pathology
Macroscopic and microscopic features
Management
Prognosis

Mnemonic

"In A Surgeon's Gown, Some Physicians Might Make Progress"

1.4 CLASSIFICATION OF SKIN GRAFTS

Split thickness	(contain varying amounts of dermis) – meshed or unmeshed
Full thickness	(contains the entire dermis)

Graft
– *Tissue separated from its donor bed and blood supply that relies on the ingrowth of new vessels for survival.*

Primary graft contraction
– *Physiological recoil of a newly harvested skin graft due to its inherent elastic properties. Full thickness skin grafts exhibit greater primary contraction than split thickness skin grafts.*

Secondary graft contraction
– *Contraction of a graft to the dimensions of the underlying wound over the period of graft maturation. Split thickness skin grafts exhibit greater secondary contraction than full thickness skin grafts. (Dermis appears to inhibit the differentiation of myofibroblasts).*

Composite graft
– *A combination of tissue types harvested in unity as a graft.*

1.5 CLASSIFICATION OF STAGES OF SPLIT SKIN GRAFT TAKE
(1) Adherence
(2) Imbibition
(3) Inosculation
(4) Revascularization

Adherence
– *Attachment of the graft to the host bed.*

Imbibition
– *Serum absorption by the graft*

Inosculation
– *Anastomoses between the graft and host vessels*

Revascularization
– *Re-establishment of a blood supply*

1.6   CLASSIFICATION OF FLAPS: "THE FIVE CS"

Adapted from Adrian Richards. Key Notes on Plastic Surgery. Blackwell Science; 2002

Circulation *("blood supply")*	– Random pattern – Axial (direct, fasciocutaneous, musculo-cutaneous, venous)
Composition *("component parts")*	– Cutaneous, fasciocutaneous, fascial, musculocutaneous, muscle, osseocuta-neous, osseous
Contiguity *("relationship to defect")*	– Local, regional, distant, free
Contouring *("type of movement")* (Figs. 1.2–1.4)	– Advancement, rotation, transposition, interpolation
Conditioning	– Delay

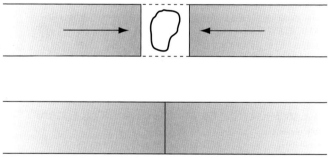

FIGURE 1.2. Bilateral advancement flaps.

Flap
– *A composite block of tissue with its own blood supply.*

Pedicled flap
– *Tissue that remains attached to its blood supply and is transferred from one part of the body to another.*

Perforator flap
– *A flap based on a visible musculocutaneous or septocutaneous perforating vessel that is dissected free from surrounding muscle to obtain the desired pedicle length.*

Flap Design

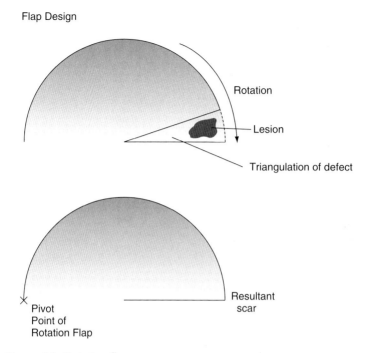

FIGURE 1.3. Rotation flap.

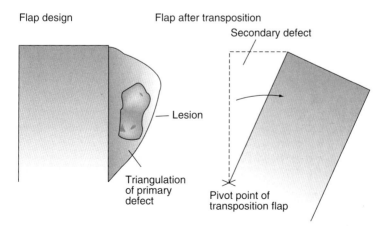

FIGURE 1.4. Transposition flap.

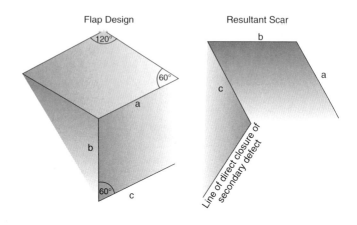

Flap Design   Resultant Scar

FIGURE 1.5. Rhomboid flap.

Free flap
– *Tissue that is transferred from one part of the body to another and is revascularized by microvascular anastomoses to recipient vessels.*

Chimeric flap
– *A flap comprising of separate components ultimately supplied by the same source vessel.*

Delay
– *A planned initial manoeuvre to partially interrupt the blood supply of a flap before moving it to a new position at a later date. This facilitates the opening up of "choke" vessels, reorientation of existing flap vessels and the sprouting of new vessels within the flap which improves the flap's ultimate blood supply.*

Crane principle
– *A technique to convert an ungraftable bed into a graftable bed. It involves transferring a flap into the defect, and after a period of time returning the superficial portion of the flap to its original position, minimizing the aesthetic defect and allowing the remaining now graftable bed to be skin grafted.*

Z-plasty
– *A technique involving the transposition of two triangular flaps, allowing elongation, realignment, and breaking up of a straight scar (Figs. 1.6–1.8)*

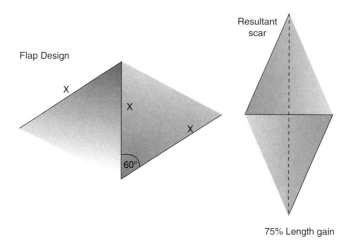

FIGURE 1.6. Classic Z-plasty.

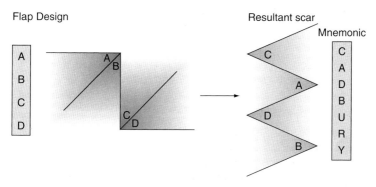

FIGURE 1.7. The 4 – Flap plasty.

1.7   CLASSIFICATION OF THEORETICAL LENGTH GAIN DEPENDING ON THE ANGLE OF DESIGN OF A Z-PLASTY

Z-plasty angle	Theoretical length gain (%)
30/30°	25
45/45°	50
60/60°	75
75/75°	100
90/90°	120

FIGURE 1.8. The 5 – Flap plasty or "Jumping Man" flap.

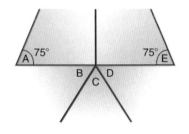

Flap design

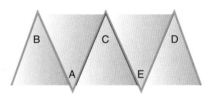

Resultant scar

1.8 CLASSIFICATION OF FASCIOCUTANEOUS FLAPS: CORMACK AND LAMBERTY (FIGURE 1.9)

Cormack GC, Lamberty BG: The Arterial Anatomy of Skin Flaps. Edinburgh, Churchill Livingstone; 1986

Blood reaches the flap from fasciocutaneous vessels running from deep arteries of the body. Most flaps raised in a limb have a fasciocutaneous pattern of blood supply.

Type A
Multiple, unnamed fasciocutaneous vessels entering the base of the flap
E.g., Ponten lower leg flaps

Type B
Single fasciocutaneous vessel running along the axis of the flap
E.g., Scapular, parascapular flaps

Type C
Multiple perforating vessels from a deep artery in the septum between muscles
E.g., Radial forearm flap

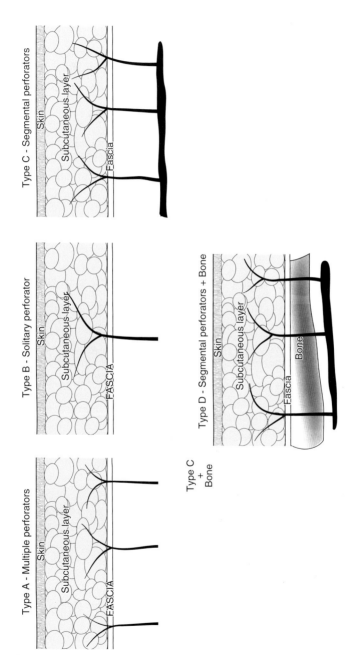

FIGURE 1.9. Classification of fasciocutaneous flaps – Cormack and Lamberty.

Type D
Type C+ Bone
E.g., Radial forearm flap with radius
Lateral arm flap with humoral lateral supracondylar ridge

1.9 CLASSIFICATION OF FASCIAL AND FASCIOCUTANEOUS FLAPS: MATHES AND NAHAI (FIGURE 1.10)

Mathes SJ, Nahai F. Reconstructive surgery: Principles, Anatomy, and Technique. New York, Churchill Livingstone; 1997

Type A	Direct cutaneous pedicle
Type B	Septocutaneous pedicle
Type C	Musculocutaneous pedicle

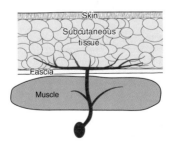

FIGURE 1.10. Classification of fascial and fasciocutaneous flaps – Mathes–Nahai.

1.10 CLASSIFICATION OF MUSCULOCUTANEOUS FLAPS: MATHES AND NAHAI (FIGURE 1.11)

Mathes SJ, Nahai F. Classification of the vascular anatomy of muscles: experimental and clinical correlation. Plast Reconstr Surg 1981;67:177

Based on perforators that reach skin through muscle

Type I
One vascular pedicle nourishes the whole flap (Gastrocnemius, Tensor fascia lata, Abductor digiti minimi)

Type II
Dominant vascular pedicle with additional minor vascular pedicles (Trapezius, Gracilis)

Type III
Two dominant vessels (Rectus abdominus, Gluteus Maximus, Serratus, Temporalis)

Type IV
Segmental supply (Sartorius, Tibialis anterior, Flexor hallucis longus)

Type V
Dominant pedicle but alternative minor pedicles which can support the flap (Latissimus Dorsi, Pectoralis Major)

1.11 CLASSIFICATION OF VENOUS FLAPS: THATTE AND THATTE (FIGURE 1.12)

Thatte MR, Thatte RL: Venous flaps. Plast Reconstr Surg 1992;91:747
A small artery may run with a vein
Flaps are based on a venous pedicle
E.g., Saphenous flap based on the short saphenous vein applied to knee defects

Type I – Single venous pedicle
Type II – Bipedicled venous flap
Type III – Arteriovenous venous flap

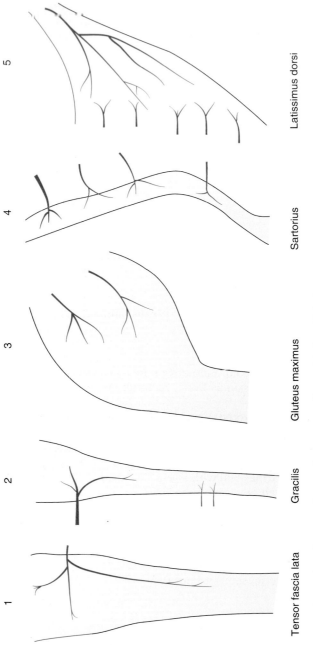

Tensor fascia lata   Gracilis   Gluteus maximus   Sartorius   Latissimus dorsi

FIGURE 1.11. Classification of musculocutaneous flaps – Mathes–Nahai.

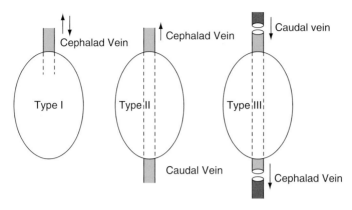

FIGURE 1.12. Classification of venous flaps – Thatte and Thatte.

1.12 CLASSIFICATION OF TYPES OF TRANSPLANT

Autograft
Allograft
Isograft
Xenograft

Heterotopic transplant
Orthotopic transplant

Autograft
– *Tissue transplanted from one site to another within the same individual*

Allograft
– *Tissue transplanted between unrelated individuals of the same species*

Isograft
– *Tissue transplanted between genetically identical individuals*

Xenograft
– *Tissue transplanted between different species*

Heterotopic transplant
– *Transplantation of tissue into an anatomically different site*

Orthotopic transplant
– *Transplantation of tissue into an anatomically similar site*

1.13   CLASSIFICATION OF TYPES OF WOUND HEALING

Primary intention
Delayed primary closure
Secondary intention

Primary intention
– *Skin edges directly apposed, normally heals well with minimal scar formation*

Delayed primary closure
– *Wound left open and closed as a secondary procedure*

Secondary intention
– *Open wound which heals by contraction and epithelialization*

1.14   CLASSIFICATION OF PHASES OF WOUND HEALING

Haemostasis
Inflammation
Proliferation
Remodelling

Wound contraction
– *A process in which the surrounding skin is pulled towards an open wound and thought to be mediated by myofibroblast activity*

Contracture
– *A pathological manifestation of wound contraction resulting in tissue shortening that compromises joint mobility and function (and potentially growth in children)*

Epithelialization
– *Migration of keratinocytes across a partial thickness wound to restore epidermal continuity*

1.15   CLASSIFICATION OF FACTORS AFFECTING WOUND HEALING

Local
Blood supply
Radiation
Infection
Trauma
Nerve injury
Foreign body
Pressure
Oedema

Systemic
Nutrition
Pharmacological – steroids, chemotherapy
Endocrine – diabetes
Medical – jaundice, uraemia, cancer
Age
Smoking
Toxins

Congenital
Ehlers Danlos, Progeria, Werners, Epidermolysis bullosa, Cutis laxa, Pseudoxanthoma elasticum

1.16 CLASSIFICATION OF TYPES OF WOUND AND ASSOCIATED INFECTION RISK

Cruse PJ, Foord R: The epidemiology of wound infection. A 10 year prospective study of 62,939 wounds. Surg Clin North Am 1980; 60(1):27–40

		Infection risk (%)
Clean	(Class I)	< 2
Clean contaminated	(Class II)	< 10
Contaminated	(Class III)	< 20
Dirty	(Class IV)	Approximately 40

1.17 CLINICAL CLASSIFICATION OF SCARS

Mustoe TA et al. International recommendations on scar management. Plas Reconstr Surg 2002;110:560–571

Mature scar
Immature scar
Linear hypertrophic
Widespread hypertrophic
Minor keloid
Major keloid

Hypertrophic scar
– *Excessive cutaneous scar formation which is contained within the borders of the original wound.*

Keloid
– *Excessive cutaneous scar formation which extends outside the borders of the original wound.*

1.18 CLASSIFICATION OF SCAR ASSESSMENT

1.18.1 Vancouver Burn Scar Assessment Scale (Summarized)
Sullivan T et al. Rating the burn scar. J Burn Care Rehabil 1990; 11:256–260

	Score
Pigmentation	0–2
Vascularity	0–3
Pliability	0–3
Height	0–3

1.18.2 Global Acne Scarring Classification
Goodman G, Baron J. The management of post acne scarring. Dermatol Surg 2007;33:1176

Grade 1	Macular	Erythematous, hyper, or hypopigmented flat marks
Grade 2	Mild	Mild rolling, small soft papular
Grade 3	Moderate	More significant rolling, shallow boxcar, mild to moderate hypertrophic or papular scars
Grade 4	Severe	Punched out atrophic (deep boxcar), ice pick, bridges and tunnels, marked atrophy, dystrophic significant hypertrophy, or keloid

1.19 CLASSIFICATION OF MUSCLE

Anatomical	(a) Striated
	(b) Smooth
Innervation	(a) Voluntary
	(b) Autonomic
Functional	Blood supply (see Mathes and Nahai classification)

1.20 CLASSIFICATION OF CARTILAGE
Hyaline
Elastic
Fibrocartilage

1.21 CLASSIFICATION OF SOURCES OF AUTOLOGOUS CARTILAGE GRAFTS

Costal cartilage
Auricular cartilage
Nasal septum

1.22 CLASSIFICATION OF BONE TYPE

Endochondral (e.g., Long bones)
Membranous (e.g., Craniofacial skeleton)

1.23 CLASSIFICATION OF PHASES OF FRACTURE HEALING

Haemostasis
Inflammation
Proliferation – periosteal/endosteal
Callus formation
Remodelling

1.24 CLASSIFICATION OF TYPES OF BONE GRAFT

Autogenous
Allogenic
Xenogeneic
Bone substitutes
 – Calcium phosphates
 – Calcium sulfate
 – Methylmethacrylate

1.25 CLASSIFICATION OF NERVE INJURY

1.25.1 Seddon 1947

Seddon H. The use of autogenous grafts for the repair of large gaps
in peripheral nerves. Br J Surg 1947; 35:151–167

Neuropraxia (equates to Sunderland 1)
Axonotmesis (equates to Sunderland 2)
Neurotmesis (equates to Sunderland 3–5)

Neuropraxia
– A temporary conduction block in a nerve with axonal continuity

Axonotmesis
*– Loss in axonal continuity. Surrounding connective tissue
 components intact*

Neurotmesis
– *Complete disruption of the axonal component as well as disruption of the surrounding sheath of connective tissue*

1.25.2 Sunderland 1951

Sunderland S. A classification of peripheral nerve injuries producing loss of function. Brain 1951;74:491–516

1 Axonal continuity, conduction impaired, segment of demyelination (should recover in 12 weeks)
2 Axonal disruption, distal Wallerian degeneration
3 Axonal/endoneurium disruption – perineurium intact – some recovery
4 Epineurium only intact – neuroma in continuity
5 Complete nerve disruption
6 Mackinnon modification – Mixed/segmental injury

Scores 4–5 require surgical intervention; 6 variable recovery

1.26 GRADING OF SENSORY RECOVERY (SUMMARY)
Mackinnon S, Dellon A. Surgery of the Peripheral Nerve. New York, Thieme; 1988

S0	No recovery
S1	Deep cutaneous sensation
S2	Superficial sensation
S2+	Hypersensitivity of superficial sensation
S3	Pain and Touch, 2 pd > 15 mm
S3+	Good localization, 2 pd 7–15 mm
S4	Complete recovery, 2 pd 2–6 mm

1.27 MRC GRADING OF MOTOR FUNCTION (SUMMARY)
Barnes R. Traction injuries of the brachial plexus in adults. J Bone Joint Surg Br 1949;31:10–36

M0	No contraction
M1	Palpable contraction
M2	Active movement of joint (gravity excluded)
M3	Active motion of joint against gravity
M4	Weaker than normal strength – full range of active motion
M5	Normal strength – full range of active motion

Nerve conduction studies
– *An electrical test which records measurements of conduction velocity along a nerve.*

Electromyography
– *An electrical test which measures motor action potentials following stimulation of a motor nerve.*

1.28 CLASSIFICATION OF NERVE FIBRE TYPE

			Conduction velocity (ms^{-1})	Diameter (μm)
Myelinated	Group A	Alpha	70–120	12–20
		Beta	60–80	10–15
		Gamma	15–40	3–8
		Delta	10–30	3–8
	(motor and sensory)			
	Group B		5–15	1–3
	(preganglionic autonomic)			
Unmyelinated	Group C		0.5–2.5	0.2–1.5
	(pain and temperature)			

Double crush phenomenon
– *Entrapment at one level associated with symptoms of compression at another level along the same nerve*

Wallerian degeneration
– *Axon and myelin degeneration and phagocytosis by Schwann cells and macrophages distal to the site of nerve injury*

Neurotrophism
– *The ability of distal receptors to enhance the maturation of nerve fibres and direct nerve regrowth in a specific direction*

Neurotropism
– *The ability of regenerating fibres to demonstrate tissue and end organ specificity*

1.29 CLASSIFICATION OF SUTURES

(a) Material	Natural	Synthetic
(b) Degradability	Absorbable	Non-absorbable
(c) Number of filaments	Braided	Monofilament

1.30 CLASSIFICATION OF IMPLANT MATERIALS

Metals	Stainless steel, titanium, gold
Ceramics	Hydroxyapatite, hydroxyapatite cement
Biologic materials	Collagen, alloderm
Polymers	Silicone, polymethlymethacrylate, polyester, polyamide, polyethylene, polypropylene

Alloplastic
– Material of synthetic origin

Autologous
– Tissue derived from self

1.31 CLASSIFICATION AND EXAMPLES OF DRESSINGS
Films (Opsite, Tegaderm)
Hydrogel sheets
Amorphous gels
Hydrocolloids (Duoderm, Granuflex)
Foams (Lyofoam)
Alginates (Kaltostat, Sorbsan)
Collagen
Contact layers
Low adherent (Paraffin gauze, Melolin)
Vacuum dressing
Biological dressing
Enzymatic dressing
Odour absorbent (Actisorb Silver)

1.32 ALPHABETICAL CLASSIFICATION OF IDEAL PROPERTIES OF DRESSINGS
"ABCDEFGHI"
O'Brien CM

Available, absorptive
Barrier (protective)
Cost effective, conformable, comfortable
Dead or necrotic material removal
Epithelialization encouraged
Granulation encouraged
Healing promoted, hydration
Flexible
non **I**rritant

1.33   CLASSIFICATION OF TISSUE EXPANDER BIOLOGY ACCORDING TO SKIN COMPONENTS

Austad ED, Paysk KA, McClatchey KD, Cherry GW. Histomorphologic evaluation of guinea pig skin and soft tissue after controlled tissue expansion. Plast Reconstr Surg 1982;70:704–710

Epidermis – Thickens (this contrasts with other components of skin)

Dermis	Thins, collagen increases
Skin appendages	Separate, altered hair density and sensation
Subcutaneous tissue	Atrophy, fibrosis
Muscle	Atrophy, increased mitochondria
Bone	Resorption and deformity
Nerve	Altered conductivity
Mitotic rate of expanded skin	Increases
Vascularity	Increases, angiogenesis secondary to ischaemia

1.34   CLASSIFICATION OF TYPES OF TISSUE EXPANDER

Shape	Oval, round, square, rectangle, croissant
Size	Base, projection
Location of port	Integrated or remote
Envelope	Smooth, textured, with differential thickening

1.35   TISSUE EXPANDER CAPSULE CLASSIFICATION – PAYSK

Inner zone	Macrophages within a layer of fibrin
Central zone	Fibroblasts, Myofibroblasts
Transitional zone	Loose fibres of collagen
Outer zone	Blood vessels and collagen

Creep
– Skin stretch in response to a sudden but constant load

Stress relaxation
– After time, a decrease occurs in the load required to maintain the same length

1.36   MICROSURGERY

Microsurgery
– Surgery with the aid of a microscope
– Greek derivation: – mikros – small
*   – skopein = to view*

Triangulation
A technique of placing sutures 120° apart at the anastomosis site (helps to avoid inadvertent inclusion of the back wall).

Reperfusion injury
Release of accumulated free radicals into the circulation following Re-establishment of a blood supply

No-reflow phenomenon
– *Lack of tissue perfusion despite adequate patent arterial and venous anastomoses. It is postulated to be due to endothelial swelling, interstitial oedema and platelet aggregation*

Ischaemic time
– *The time interval between interrupting and re-establishing a blood supply*

1.37 CLASSIFICATION OF TYPES OF MICROVASCULAR ANASTOMOSIS
End to end
End to side
Sleeve (one end inside the other)

1.38 CLASSIFICATION OF FLAP MONITORING METHODS
Clinical examination
Ultrasound Doppler
Laser Doppler
Thermocouple probes
Photoplethysmography
Transcutaneous oxygen monitoring
pH monitoring
Intravenous fluorescein
Near infrared spectroscopy

1.39 CLASSIFICATION OF TECHNICAL REASONS FOR FLAP FAILURE
(Any manoeuvre which produces intimal damage predisposes to thrombosis)

Suture technique	– loose, tight, too many, tension, unequal spacing, partial thickness bites
Vessel	– rough dissection, desiccation, diathermy, prolonged vasospasm
Clamp pressure	> 30 g mm^{-2}
Needle	– calibre too large, repeated stabs

1.40 VIRCHOW'S TRIAD

Factors initially thought to contribute to venous thrombosis but now applied to the arterial circulation

Stasis
Endothelial damage
Hypercoagulability

1.41 ACLAND'S CLASSIFICATION OF FACTORS INFLUENCING PATENCY OF AN ANASTOMOSIS

Surgical precision
Vessel diameter
Blood flow
Tension
Anticoagulant/antithrombolytic agents

1.42 OPTIONS FOR FLAP VIABILITY IMPROVEMENT: CLASSIFICATION OF INTERVENTION

Preoperative	Planning, theatre set up, patient selection and optimization
Preanastomosis	Delay, flap hypothermia (reduce metabolic rate), short ischaemic time, anaesthetic input
Postanastomosis	Patient – Keep warm, well hydrated, pain free Leeches Drugs – Steroids, aspirin, dextran, heparin

1.43 LOCAL ANAESTHETICS: CLASSIFICATION ACCORDING TO STRUCTURE

Amino amide (lidocaine, prilocaine, bupivacaine)
– Metabolized in the liver, excreted by the kidney

Amino ester (procaine, cocaine, benzocaine, amethocaine)
– Hydrolysis in plasma by pseudocholinesterase, unstable in solution and may cause allergic reactions

1.44 LOCAL ANAESTHETICS: CLASSIFICATION ACCORDING TO LENGTH OF ACTION

Doses	Plain	With adrenaline	Duration (min)
Lignocaine	3 mg kg^{-1}	7 mg kg^{-1}	60–120
Bupivacaine	2–3 mg kg^{-1}	3 mg kg^{-1}	240–480

1% solution = 10 mg ml^{-1}
EMLA: Eutectic mixture of local anaesthetics – 2.5% prilocaine and
2.5% lignocaine

1.45 AMERICAN SOCIETY OF ANESTHESIOLOGISTS' PHYSICAL STATUS CLASSIFICATION (ASA GRADE)

Class I	No systemic disease
Class II	Mild to moderate systemic disease – no functional limitation
Class III	Severe systemic disease with functional limitation
Class IV	Severe systemic disease that is life-threatening
Class V	Moribund patient
E	Emergency surgery

1.46 LASER
LASER
– Light amplification by stimulated emission of radiation

Selective photothermolysis
– Selective damage of target tissue rather than surrounding normal tissue by the preferential absorption of light of a particular wavelength when delivered to the target during a pulse duration less than or equal to the thermal relaxation time of the target. (theory described by Anderson and Parrish 1983).

Thermal relaxation time
– Time taken for a given volume of tissue to cool to 50% of the initial temperature.

Energy
– Proportional to number of photons (J)

Power
– Rate of delivery of energy (W or J s^{-1})

Power density
= power/spot

Fluence
= power/spot/time (J cm^{-2})

1.47 CLASSIFICATION OF CLASSES OF LASER
(British Standard on Laser Safety BS EN 60825–1: 1994 as amended)

Class 1	Power output is below the level required to cause eye injury
	The irradiance does not exceed the maximum permissible exposure
	Lasers of a higher class may be incorporated into this group if the beam is protected from access by adequate engineering (laser printer)
Class 1M	Highly divergent or large diameter beam (fibre–optic communication)
Class 2	Blinking response prevents eye damage on exposure to beam
	Beam wavelength between 400 and 700 nm
	Maximum power output 1 mW (laser pointer, barcode scanner)
Class 2M	Highly divergent beam
	Beam wavelength between 400 and 700 nm
	Maximum power output 1 mW (civil engineering orientation or level instruments)
Class 3R	Potential to cause eye injury
	Maximum power output 5 mW
Class 3B	Potential to cause eye injury from direct beam and reflection
	Power output up to 500 mW (research lasers)
Class 4	Capable of causing injury to eye or skin
	Power output >500 mW
	Fire or flume hazard (laser surgery, laser displays, metal cutting lasers)

1.48   CLASSIFICATION OF LASER APPLICATIONS IN PLASTIC SURGERY

Skin lesions – congenital and acquired
Tattoo removal
Skin resurfacing
Hair removal

1.49   HAIR

1.49.1   Histological Classification of Parts of a Hair Follicle

Infundibulum
Isthmus
Stern
Bulb

1.49.2   Classification of Hair Growth Phases
Anagen – Growth phase
Catagen – Transition phase
Telogen – Resting phase

1.49.3   Classification of Hair Removal Techniques
Plucking
Shaving
Waxing
Depilatory creams
Electrolysis
LASER

1.49.4   Classification of Scalp Alopecia
McCauley RL, Oliphant JR, Robson MC. Ann Plast Surg 1990;25(2): 103–115

Type I   Single alopecia segment
           (a) < 25% – single expander
           (b) 25–50% – single expander/over-inflation
           (c) 50–75% – multiple expanders
           (d) >75% – multiple expanders (uniform alopecia)

Type II   Multiple areas of alopecia amenable to tissue expansion (segmental alopecia)

Type III   Multiple areas of alopecia not amenable to tissue expansion (patchy alopecia)

Type IV   Total alopecia

Tumour
– *An abnormal mass of tissue the growth of which exceeds and is uncoordinated with that of normal tissue and persists in the same injurious manner after cessation of the stimulus*

Ulcer
– *A breach in the epithelium with one or more factors preventing it from healing*

Apoptosis
– Programmed cell death

1.50 WHO CLASSIFICATION OF BODY MASS INDEX

<18.5 kg m^{-2}	Underweight, thin
18.5–24.9 kg m^{-2}	Healthy weight, healthy
25.0–29.9 kg m^{-2}	Grade I Obesity, overweight
30.0–39.9 kg m^{-2}	Grade II Obesity, obesity
>40 kg m^{-2}	Grade III Obesity, morbid obesity

Body mass index
$$\frac{\textit{Weight (in kg)}}{\textit{Height (in m}^2)}$$

Sensitivity
Proportion of reference test positive (diseased) subjects who test positive with the screening test (i.e., "True positives")

Specificity
Proportion of reference test negative (healthy) subjects who test negative with the screening test (i.e., "True negatives")

Chapter 2
Hand Surgery

2.1 CLASSIFICATION SYSTEMS OF CONGENITAL HAND DEFORMITY
Morphology based
Embryology based
Genetic based (gene localization)

2.2 CLASSIFICATION OF CONGENITAL LIMB MALFORMATIONS
Swanson A. A classification for congenital limb malformation. *J Hand Surg* 1976; 1:8

Accepted by the American Society for Surgery of the Hand (ASSH) and the International Federation of Societies for Surgery of the Hand (IFSSH).

This is the most commonly used system

2.2.1 Overview
I.   Failure of formation of parts
II.   Failure of differentiation of parts
III. Duplication
IV.   Overgrowth
V.   Undergrowth
VI.   Congenital constriction ring syndromes
VII. Generalized skeletal abnormalities

Mary O'Brien, *Plastic and Hand Surgery in Clinical Practice,*
DOI: 10.1007/978-1-84800-263-0_2,
© Springer-Verlag London Limited 2009

2.2.2 Sub-classifications for Each Group

Failure of Formation of Parts Sub-classifications

(A) Transverse

(B) Longitudinal – Radial longitudinal deficiency (RLD), Central deficiency, Ulnar longitudinal deficiency
– Intercalated (Phocomelia)

Radial longitudinal deficiency (also known as "Radial Club Hand")

– *Hypoplasia or absence of the radius and or radial structures resulting in radial deviation. The wrist is unstable. It may be associated with other abnormalities. (associated syndromes include VATER, Holt Oram, TAR, Fanconi's anaemia)*

VATER syndrome
– *Vertebral anomalies, Anal atresia, Tracheo-Eesophageal fistula, Renal abnormalities +RLD*

Holt Oram syndrome
– *Cardiac abnormalities + RLD*

TAR
– *Thrombocytopenia + Absent radius*

Fanconi syndrome
– *Progressive pancytopenia, predisposition to malignancy + RLD*

Radial Longitudinal Deficiency Radiological Classification
I.   Deficient distal radial epiphysis
II. Hypoplasia of radius
III. Partial aplasia of radius
IV. Total aplasia of radius

Cleft Hand Classification
Typical
– V-shaped defect, Bilateral, Familial, Syndactyly, Cleft feet, Absence of central metacarpal shafts

Atypical (symbrachydactyly)
– U-shaped defect, Unilateral, Non-familial, No foot involvement

Ulnar longitudinal deficiency (also known as "Ulnar club hand")
 – *A congenital deficiency on the ulnar side of the hand and forearm with varying degrees of elbow dysfunction. The wrist is stable.*

Ulnar Longitudinal Deficiency: Bayne's Classification
Bayne, L. Ulnar Club Hand. In Green D, ed. *Operative Hand Surgery*. New York: Churchill Livingstone; 1982
I   Hypoplasia of ulnar
II   Partial aplasia of ulnar
III   Total aplasia of ulnar
IV   Radiohumeral synostosis

Phocomelia
 – *A congenital intercalated deficiency usually characterized by reduced numbers and function of digital skeletal elements resulting in a significantly shortened limb.*

Phocomelia Classification
1. Complete (no arm or forearm, hand attached to trunk)
2. Proximal (no arm, forearm attaches to trunk)
3. Distal (no forearm, hand attaches to humerus)

2.2.3   Failure of Differentiation of Parts Sub-classifications

Soft tissue	Bone
Syndactyly	Clinodactyly
Camptodactyly	Symphalangism
Trigger thumb	Radioulnar synostosis
Clasped thumb	Arthrogryposis
	Windblown hand

Syndactyly
 – *Digits that are joined together as a result of failure of apoptosis (programmed cell death) in that region.*

Syndactyly Classification
Complete –Fusion of affected digits to level of distal phalanx
Incomplete – Fusion proximal to level of distal phalanx but distal to mid proximal phalanx
Simple – Soft tissue involvement only
Complex – Bone in addition to soft tissue involvement
Complicated (Acrosyndactyly) – Distal bony fusion associated with proximal fenestrations (Fig. 2.1)

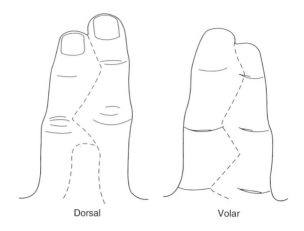

Dorsal   Volar

FIGURE 2.1. Complete, simple syndactyly release.

Acrosyndactyly Classification: Walsh
Walsh RJ. Acrosyndactyly: a study of 27 patients. *Clin Orthop* 1970;71:99–111

Moderate – Two phalanges and one interphalangeal joint per digit
Severe – One phalanx per digit

Classification of Hand Deformities Associated with Apert's Syndrome
Type I   – Central digital mass, thumb and little finger free (spade hand)
Type II   – Thumb only free (mitten/spoon hand)
Type III – Thumb and digital mass share a common nail (rose-bud/hoof hand)

Classification of Poland's Syndrome Deformities
(A) Upper limb related
  – Shortened digits (absent middle phalanx)
  – Complete simple syndactyly
  – Hand hypoplasia
  – Absent sternocostal head of the ipsilateral pectoralis major
  – Absent pectoralis minor

(B) Other associations
  – Breast and nipple hypoplasia
  – Absent anterior axillary fold
  – Absent latissimus dorsi, deltoid, serratus anterior
  – Bony abnormalities of chest wall
  – Dextrocardia

Camptodactyly
– *A congenital flexion deformity of the PIPJ that most commonly affects the little finger and is commonly bilateral.*

Camptodactyly Classification
Infant type:
Camptodactyly evident in infancy and affects both sexes equally

Adolescent type:
Camptodactyly which presents in adolescence and more commonly affects females

Camptodactyly Radiological Features Classification
1. Proximal phalanx neck indentation (from anterior lip on the base of the flexed middle phalanx)
2. Middle phalanx – wide base (antero-posteriorly), articular surface indentation
3. Proximal phalanx – flattened head (dorsal 1/3)

Trigger thumb
– *Inability to extend the thumb often associated with a nodule (Notta's node) on the flexor surface of the tendon at the level of the A1 pulley.*

Clasped thumb
– *A thumb characteristically held in adduction to the palm and extreme flexion of the MCPJ.*

Clasped Thumb Classification (Weckesser et al.)
Weckesser E, Reed J, Heiple K. Congenital clasped thumb (congenital flexion adduction deformity of the thumb). *J Bone Joint Surg* 1968;37A:1417–1428

Group I – Deficient extension but no contracture
Group II – Deficient extension, flexion contracture
Group III – Deficient extension, hypoplasia of thumb
Group IV – Miscellaneous

Clasped Thumb Classification (McCarroll)
McCarroll HR Jr. Congenital flexion deformities of the thumb. *Hand Clin* 1985;1:567–575

Supple – weak or absent thumb extensors
Complex – above + joint, ligament, muscle and skin abnormalities

Clinodactyly
- *A congenital radial or ulnar deviation of a digit most commonly seen as radial deviation of the little finger at the DIPJ due to a delta phalanx formed from a C shaped epiphysis (otherwise known as a longitudinal bracketed diaphysis).*

Clinodactyly Classification
Type 1 – Angulation minor, Phalangeal length normal
Type 2 – Angulation minor, Phalangeal length short (Down's Syndrome)
Type 3 – Marked angulation, delta phalanx

Clinodactyly Treatment Option Classification
None
Closing wedge osteotomy   – Type 1 deformity
Opening wedge osteotomy   – Type 2 deformity
Exchange wedge osteotomy
Excision of additional delta phalanx, ligament preservation:
    – Longer digit than normal
    – Triphalangeal thumb
Physiolysis – for restoration of alignment, length, and orientation

Kirner's deformity
- *Curvature of the distal phalanx of the little finger in a radial and palmar direction. Presents most commonly in females age 7–14 years*

Symphalangism
- *A failure of interphalangeal joint differentiation leading to stiff, short digits. Absent flexor and extensor tendons and absent skin creases.*

Symphalangism Classification
Hereditary
Non-hereditary (associated with syndactyly, Apert's syndrome, Poland's syndrome)

Synostosis
- *A complete or partial abnormal fusion of two bones*

Radioulnar Synostosis Classification
Primary   – absent radial head, extensive bony synostosis
Secondary – normally shaped radial head, often dislocated

Arthrogryposis multiplex congenita
– *Greek derivation meaning "curved joint"*
– *Congenital contractures in more than two joints and multiple body areas. The primary abnormality is muscular resulting in secondary joint deformity.*

Classification of Arthrogryposis (Mennen)
Loose type
Stiff type

Classification of Arthrogryposis (Weeks)
Weeks PM, Surgical correction of upper extremity deformities in arthrogrypotics. *Plastic Reconstr Surg* 1965;36:459–465

1. Single localized deformity
2. Full expression
3. Full expression + polydactyly, other systems involved in addition to neuro-musculoskeletal system

Windblown hand
– *A rare congenital condition resulting in ulnar deviation of the fingers which is progressive and commonly bilateral. It may be associated with MCPJ flexion and a first web space contracture.*

2.2.4   Duplication Sub-classifications

Types of duplication
Radial, central, ulnar, ulnar dimelia

Thumb duplication classification – Wassell
Wassell HD. The results of surgery for polydactyly of the thumb. *Clin Orthop* 1969;64:175–193

Type 1. Bifid distal phalanx
Type 2. Duplication starting at the DIPJ
Type 3. Bifid proximal phalanx
Type 4. Duplication starting at the MCPJ (commonest)
Type 5. Bifid metacarpal
Type 6. Duplication starting at the CMCJ
Type 7. Thumb duplication with a triphalangeal thumb

Bilhaut – Cloquet Procedure
– *A procedure undertaken to correct thumb duplication by sharing tissue from each thumb to create a single thumb*

Modified Bilhaut – Cloquet Procedure
  – *A tissue sharing procedure to create a single thumb from a duplication using the entire nail from one thumb to avoid residual nail deformity*

Triphalangeal thumb
  – *A thumb with an additional phalanx between the proximal and distal phalanges*

Classification of Types of Triphalangeal Thumb
(A) Delta phalanx
(B) Short rectangular phalanx
(C) Normal length rectangular phalanx

Buck-Gramcko Classification of Triphalangeal Thumbs
Buck-Gramcko D. Triphalangeal Thumb. In: *Congenital Malformations of the Hand and Forearm.* New York: Churchill Livingstone; 1998

Type I	– Rudimentary phalanx
Type II	– Short triangular middle phalanx
Type III	– Trapezoidal middle phalanx
Type IV	– Long rectangular middle phalanx
Type V and VI	– Hypoplastic triphalangeal thumb
Type VI	– Triphalangism associated with thumb polydactyly

Stelling's Classification of Polydactyly
Type I – Extra "digit" with attachment by soft tissue only (no bone)
Type II – Extra digit with all normal components articulating with a phalanx or metacarpal
Type III – Extra digit articulating with an extra metacarpal

2.2.5 Overgrowth
Macrodactyly
  – *A congenital localized hamartomatous enlargement of a digit*

True macrodactyly
  – *A localized enlargement of all structures within a digit*

Classification of Macrodactyly
Static – enlarged digit grows in proportion with the body
Progressive – enlarged digit grows progressively out of proportion with the body

Histological Classification of Macrodactyly

Type 1 – Lipofibromatous hamartomas (fat)

Type 2 – Neurofibromatosis (nerve)

Type 3 – Hyperostosis (skeletal and soft tissue, no neural association)

2.2.6 Undergrowth

Classification of Thumb Hypoplasia (Blauth)

Blauth W. Der hypoplastische daumen. *Arch Orthop Trauma Surg* 1967;62:225

This classification is based on skeletal appearance.

Grade I	Small thumb, all components present
	Bone – normal skeleton
Grade II	Small thumb
	Bone – normal skeleton
	Muscle – hypoplastic thenar muscles
	Ligament – lax UCL of MCPJ
	Adducted first web space
Grade III	Bone – skeletal hypoplasia
	Muscle – absent thenar muscles
	Tendon – abnormal extrinsics
Grade IV	Pouce flottant "floating thumb" attached by a skin bridge
Grade V	Absent thumb

Paul Smith Modification of Blauth's Classification of Thumb Hypoplasia

Smith P. *Lister's The Hand, Diagnosis and Indications*, 4th edn. London: Churchill Livingstone; 2002:505

Grade II A	Normal skeleton, MCPJ uniaxial instability
Grade II B	Thin skeleton, MCPJ multiaxial instability

Manske Modification of Blauth's Classification of Thumb Hypoplasia

Manske PR. Classification and techniques in thumb hypoplasia. In: Safar P, Amadio PC, Foucher G, eds. *Current Practice in Hand Surgery*. London: Martin Dunitz; 1977:367–370

Grade III A	Metacarpal length – normal; CMCJ – normal
Grade III B	Metacarpal – absent proximally

2.2.7 Congenital Constriction Band Syndrome (Congenital Ring Constriction)

Congenital constriction band syndrome:

– *Tight bands arising in utero, which involve either partially or completely part of the limb.*

Patterson's Classification of Congenital Ring Constrictions

Patterson TJS. Congenital ring constrictions. *Br J Plastic Surg* 1961;14:1–31

1. Simple soft tissue constriction (groove)
2. Constriction associated with distal deformity (+/– lymphoedema)
3. Constriction associated with acrosyndactyly (fusion of distal parts)

    I   Tips joined

    II   Tips joined
           Web creep

    III   Tips joined
           No web
           Complete syndactyly
           Proximal sinus

4. Constriction resulting in autoamputation

2.2.8   Generalized Skeletal Abnormality

GENERAL HAND CLASSIFICATION SYSTEMS

2.3 ANATOMICAL CLASSIFICATION BY ZONE OF EXTENSOR TENDON INJURY (FIG. 2.2)

Zones in the digit

Zone I	Overlying DIPJ
II	Between PIPJ and DIPJ
III	Overlying PIPJ
IV	Between MCPJ and PIPJ
V	Overlying MCPJ
VI	Between extensor retinaculum and MCPJ
VII	Under extensor retinaculum
VIII	Proximal to extensor retinaculum

(In the finger even numbers are over bone, odd numbers over a joint)

Zones in the thumb

I	Overlying IPJ
II	Overlying proximal phalanx
III	Overlying MCPJ
IV	Overlying metacarpal
V	Overlying carpus

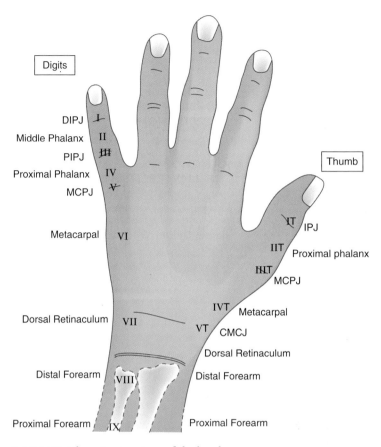

FIGURE 2.2. The extensor zones of the hand.

2.3.1 Extensor Compartments
1. APL/EPB   (a longus and a brevis)
2. ECRL/ECRB   (a longus and a brevis)
3. EPL
4. EIP/EDC
5. EDM
6. ECU

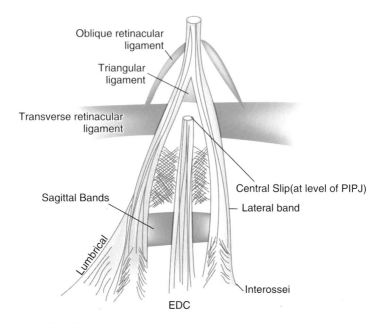

Oblique retinacular ligament

Triangular ligament

Transverse retinacular ligament

Central Slip(at level of PIPJ)

Sagittal Bands

Lateral band

Lumbrical

Interossei

EDC

FIGURE 2.3. Diagram of an extensor tendon.

2.4 FLEXOR TENDON INJURY ZONES: VERDAN

Verdan C. Half a century of flexor tendon surgery. *J Bone Joint Surg* 1972;54A:472 (Fig. 2.4)

Zone
1. Distal to FDS insertion (therefore includes FDP alone)
2. Proximal A1 pulley to FDS insertion ("No man's land" – Bunnell)
3. Distal margin of carpal tunnel to just proximal to A1 pulley
4. Within the carpal tunnel "Enemy territory"
5. Distal forearm musculotendinous junctions to proximal carpal tunnel

Thumb Zones
1. Distal to IPJ
2. Overlying proximal phalanx, i.e., A1 pulley to IPJ
3. Thenar eminence
4. and 5. As above

2.5 TENDON HEALING CLASSIFICATIONS

– Classification according to mechanism of tendon healing
  Extrinsic healing
  Intrinsic healing

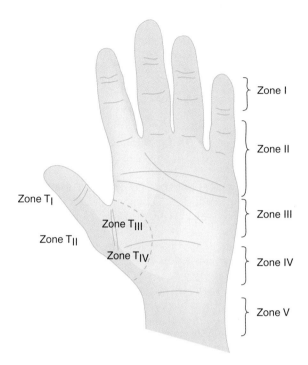

FIGURE 2.4. Flexor tendon zones of the hand.

– Classification according to phases of tendon healing
  Inflammation
  Proliferation
  Remodelling

2.6 CLOSED AVULSION OF FDP: LEDDY AND PACKER
Leddy JP, Packer JW. Avulsion of the profundus tendon in athletes.
J Hand Surg 1977;2-A:66–69

1. Tendon retracts into palm, both vinculae also ruptured
2. Distal tendon held by long vinculum at level of PIPJ
3. Fracture fragment large trapped at level of A4 pulley
   Tendon unable to retract further

Rugby finger
*Lunn PG, Lamb DW.Rugby finger – avulsion of profundus of ring
finger. J Hand Surg (Br) 1984;9(1):69–71*
– Avulsion of the profundus tendon of the ring finger

Stener Lesion

Stener B. Displacement of the ruptured ulnar collateral ligament of the MCPJ of the thumb. J Bone Joint Surg 1962;44B:869–879

– A traumatic disruption of the UCL of the thumb at the MCPJ resulting in the torn ligament lying superficial to the adductor expansion thus preventing healing

Mallet finger

– An extension lag at the DIPJ associated with loss of active DIPJ extension

2.7 DOYLE'S CLASSIFICATION OF MALLET FINGER INJURY

Doyle JR. Extensor tendons – acute injuries. In: Green DP, ed. *Operative Hand Surgery*, vol. 2, 3 edn. New York: Churchill-Livingstone; 1993:1925–1954

Type 1   Closed injury +/– avulsion fracture (most common type)
Type 2   Open injury, laceration at or proximal to DIPJ, loss of tendon continuity
Type 3   Open injury + soft tissue and tendon loss
Type 4   A Transepiphyseal plate fracture
         B Fracture 20–50% articular surface (hyperflexion injury)
         C Fracture > 50% articular surface, volar subluxation (hyperextension injury)

2.8 CLASSIFICATION OF AETIOLOGY OF A FLEXION CONTRACTURE (LIMITATION OF EXTENSION)

Smith P, ed. *Lister's The Hand, Diagnosis and Indications*. London: Churchill Livingstone; 2002:179

Extensor laceration
Bony block
Collateral adhesions
Palmar plate shortening
Flexor tendon shortened, adhesions
Sheath involved in Dupuytren's contracture
Skin scar contracture

2.8.1   Classification of Aetiology of an Extension Contracture (Limitation of Flexion)

Smith P, ed. *Lister's The Hand, Diagnosis and Indications*. London: Churchill Livingstone; 2002:181

Skin scar contracture, skin loss
Extensor long, intrinsic contracture
Capsule adhesions

Collateral adhesions
Bony block
Chondral fractures
Palmar plate
Flexor tendon adherence within sheath
Oedema

2.9 NERVE INJURY CLASSIFICATION SYSTEMS

See Chapter 1 – Fundamentals of Plastic Surgery Classifications
and Definitions

2.9.1 Classification of Types of Nerve Injury

It may be classified according to mechanism of injury:

- Laceration
- Avulsion
- Compression
- Traction
- Abnormal excursion
- Tethering
- Ischaemia
- Vibration

2.9.2 Brachial Plexus Injury: Millesi

Millesi H. Surgical management of brachial plexus injuries.
J Hand Surg 1977;2:367–379

I   Supraganglionic
II   Infraganglionic
III Trunk
IV   Cord

2.10 ROLLING BELT INJURY

Ada et al. Rolling belt injuries in children. *J Hand Surg*
1994;19B:601–603

I   Skin lesion
II A   Skin, tendon, artery and nerve uninjured, Circulation present
II B   Skin, tendon, artery and nerve uninjured, Circulation absent
III A Skin, tendon, artery and nerve injured, Circulation present
III B Skin, tendon, artery and nerve injured, Circulation absent
IV   Total finger amputation

2.11 CLASSIFICATION OF VESSEL INJURY

(A) Complete division

Less blood loss due to contraction of muscle in the arterial wall which closes the lumen at each end of the divided vessel

(B) Partial division

Contraction of muscle maintains an opening in the vessel wall in a partial division

2.12 RING AVULSION INJURY: URBANIAK'S CLASSIFICATION

Urbaniak JR, Evans JP, Bright DS. Microvascular management of ring avulsion injuries. *J Hand Surg (Am)* 1981;6:25–30

Class I	Circulation adequate
Class II	Circulation inadequate: vessel repair preserves viability
Class III	Complete degloving or amputation

2.12.1 Ring Avulsion Injury: Kay's Classification

Kay S, Werntz J, Wolff TW. Ring avulsion injuries: classification and prognosis. *J Hand Surg* 1989;14A:204–213

Class I	Circulation adequate + /– skeletal injury
Class II	Circulation inadequate (arterial and venous), no skeletal injury
	(a) Arterial circulation inadequate only
	(b) Venous circulation inadequate only
Class III	Circulation inadequate (arterial and venous) fracture or joint injury present
Class IV	Complete amputation

2.13 CLASSIFICATION OF REPLANTATION

Macroreplant

– Amputate has high muscle bulk. Speed important to prevent reperfusion injury

Microreplant

– Amputate is usually a digit. Longer ischaemic time

2.14 CLASSIFICATION OF THUMB AMPUTATION AND RECONSTRUCTIVE OPTIONS

Kleinman and Strickland. Thumb reconstruction. In: *Green's Operative Hand Surgery*. New York: Churchill Livingstone; 1999: 2096 (Fig. 2.5)

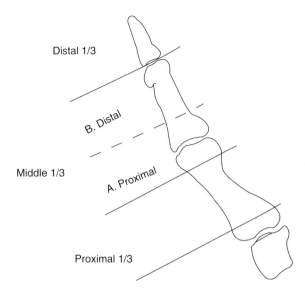

Distal 1/3

B. Distal

Middle 1/3

A. Proximal

Proximal 1/3

FIGURE 2.5. Levels of thumb amputation.

Proximal third		–Pollicization
Middle third		
	A. Proximal	–Toe to thumb
		–Osteoplastic reconstruction
		–Dorsal rotation flap
	B. Distal	–Web deepening
		–Metacarpal lengthening
		–Toe to thumb
Distal third		–Primary closure
		–Toe to thumb
		–Local flaps

2.14.1   Levels of Thumb Amputation
Morrison W, O'Brien BM, Macleod AM. Experience with thumb reconstruction. *Br J Hand Surg* 1984;9:224

Total	Level of MCPJ
Proximal subtotal	Midshaft proximal phalanx
Distal subtotal	Base of distal phalanx
Soft tissue or segmental	

2.15 EPIPHYSEAL FRACTURES: SALTER AND HARRIS CLASSIFICATION

Salter RB, Harris WR. Injuries involving the epiphyseal plate. *J Bone Joint Surg* 1963;45A:587–622 (Fig. 2.6)

Type I   Shearing of epiphysis from metaphysis
Type II   Epiphysis separated taking a small fragment of metaphysis
Type III   Epiphysis intra-articular fracture. No interference with epiphyseal plate
Type IV   Vertical displaced fracture through epiphysis, growth plate, and metaphysis
Type V   Compression fracture. No evident injury of epiphysis or metaphysis

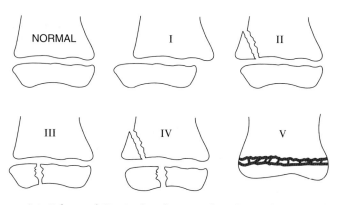

FIGURE 2.6. Salter and Harris classification of epiphyseal fractures.

2.16 CLASSIFICATION OF LONG BONE FRACTURE PATTERNS

Head   Condylar, T shape
Diaphysis   Spiral
             Longitudinal
             Oblique
             Transverse
             Comminuted
Base   Palmar
             Dorsal
             Lateral
Physis   See above Salter–Harris classification

2.17 SCAPHOID FRACTURE CLASSIFICATION—HERBERT CLASSIFICATION

A	Acute, stable	A_1 Tubercle A_2 Nondisplaced crack in waist
B	Acute, unstable	B_1 Oblique, distal third B_2 Displaced or Mobile Waist B_3 Proximal Pole B_4 Fracture dislocation B_5 Comminuted
C	Delayed Union	
D	Established non union	D_1 Fibrous D_2 Sclerotic

2.17.1 Scaphoid Fracture Classification–Russe Classification

Russe O. Fracture of the carpal navicular. Diagnosis, non-operative treatment, and operative treatment. *J. Bone Joint Surg* 1960;42A: 759–768

Horizontal oblique: Stable
Transverse: Stable
Vertical oblique: Unstable
Stability also depends on comminution and other factors

2.17.2 Classification of Scaphoid Nonunion

Alnot JY. Fractures et pseudarthroses du scaphoïde carpien. *Rev Chir Orthop* 1988;74:714

I   Linear pseudarthrosis
IIA   Slight resorption of bone, no displacement
IIB   Unstable pseudarthrosis, anterior flexion and bone loss, DISI (adaptive)
IIIA   Radioscaphoid arthritis
IIIB   Radiocarpal arthritis

Preiser's Disease:
– *Avascular necrosis of the scaphoid without prior injury*

Kienbock's Disease (lunatomalacia):
– *Avascular necrosis of the lunate leading to collapse*

2.18 STAGE OF KIENBOCK'S DISEASE (LICHTMAN)

Stage I   X-ray normal, bone scan increased uptake, tender lunate
Stage II   Sclerosis, no collapse
Stage III   Collapse and fragmentation of lunate
              A. Scaphoid normal alignment
              B. Scaphoid-rotatory malalignment (ring sign)
Stage IV   Perilunate arthritis, secondary degenerative changes of
              carpus

2.19 SCAPHOLUNATE ADVANCED COLLAPSE (SLAC) WRIST
Krakauer et al. *JHS* 1994;19A:751

I   Degenerative change involving radial styloid alone
II   Scaphoid fossa involvement
III   Capitolunate joint involvement

Terry Thomas Sign:
- *Increased space between the scaphoid and lunate on a postero-anterior radiograph and indicates scapholunate instability (name derived from an English actor renowned for the gap between his front teeth)*

2.20 CLASSIFICATION OF TYPES OF ARTHRITIS

Inflammatory – Rheumatoid, Psoriatic, Gout
Degenerative – Osteoarthritis
Infective   – Septic arthritis

Rheumatoid Arthritis
- *A systemic chronic inflammatory disease involving synovium of joints and tendons, characterized by inflammation and synovial proliferation*
- *It is a multi-organ disease with extra-articular manifestations*

2.20.1 Diagnostic Criteria for Rheumatoid Arthritis
Arnett FC, Edworthy SM, Bloch DA et al. The American Rheumatism Association 1987 revised criteria for the classification of rheumatoid arthritis. *Arthritis Rheum* 1988;31(3):315–324

1. Morning stiffness: lasting 1 h, located around joints
2. Three or more joint areas
3. Hand
4. Symmetric
5. Rheumatoid nodules
6. Rheumatoid factor

7. X-ray changes

Criteria 1–4 must be present for 6 weeks

4 out of 7 criteria needed for diagnosis

2.20.2 Classification of Typical Radiological Changes of Rheumatoid Arthritis

Narrow joint space

Marginal erosions

Osteoporosis

Cyst formation

Swelling of soft tissue

2.20.3 Radiological Classification of Rheumatoid Arthritis: Larsen's Grading System

Larsen. *Acta Radiol Diagn* 1977;18:481–491

0. Normal
1. Osteoporosis, swelling of soft tissue
2. Erosions, normal architecture
3. Erosions, abnormal architecture
4. Severe destruction of joint, joint line visible
5. Mutilans, joint line not visible

2.20.4 Classification of Rheumatoid Arthritis by Pathology

Proliferation

Destruction

Reparation

2.20.5 Classification of Rheumatoid Arthritis by Clinical Course

Monocyclic (one episode)

Polycyclic (multiple episodes)

Progressive (chronic deterioration)

2.20.6 Classification of Rheumatoid Arthritis by Number of Joints Involved

Monoarthropathy (single joint involvement)

Pauciarthropathy (2–4 joints involved)

Polyarthropathy (> 4 joints involved)

2.20.7 Classification Rheumatoid Arthritis by Grade of Function

Grade 1 No functional incapacity

Grade 2 Performs all tasks except the heaviest

Grade 3 Performs light tasks only

Grade 4 Chair/Bed bound

2.20.8 Classification of Neural Deficit in Atlanto-Axial Subluxation

Hospital for Special Surgery in New York; Ranawat CS, O'Leary P, Pellicci P et al. Cervical spine fusion in rheumatoid arthritis. *J Bone Joint Surg* 1979;61A:1003–1010

I	Nil
II	Subjective weakness, hyperreflexia, dysaethesia
IIIa	Objective long tract signs
IIIb	Quadriparesis

Swan neck deformity: A deformity characterized by PIPJ hyperextension and DIPJ flexion

2.20.9 Classification of Types of Swan Neck Deformity: Nalebuff

Nalebuff EA. The rheumatoid swan neck deformity. *Hand Clin* 1989;5:203–214

Type I	Full PIPJ flexion
Type II	Intrinsic tightness but full passive correction
Type III	PIPJ fixed in hyperextension
Type IV	PIPJ fixed in hyperextension, Joint destruction

2.20.10 Classification of Types of Swan Neck Deformity: Welsh and Hastings

Welsh RP, Hastings DE. Swan neck deformity in rheumatoid arthritis. *Hand* 1977;9:109–116

Type I	Secondary to primary PIPJ disease	(a) Mobile	(b) Snapping	(c) Fixed
Type II	Secondary to MCPJ disease	(a) Mobile	(b) Snapping	(c) Fixed

Boutonniere deformity:
A deformity characterized by PIPJ flexion and DIPJ extension

2.20.11 Classification of the Stages of Boutonniere Deformity: Nalebuff and Millender

Nalebuff EA, Millender LH. Surgical treatment of the boutonniere deformity in rheumatoid arthritis. *Orthop Clin North Am* 1975;6:753–763

Stage I	Extensor lag at PIPJ, Passively correctable
Stage II	40° flexion deformity at PIPJ, Passively correctable
Stage III	Fixed flexion deformity at PIPJ, Possible intraarticular damage

2.20.12 Classification of Severity of Boutonniere Deformity
Grade 1   Mild (10–15° lag)
Grade 2   Moderate (30–40° lag)
Grade 3   Severe, extension deficit

2.20.13 Classification of the Rheumatoid Thumb Deformity
Nalebuff EA. Diagnosis, classification and management of rheumatoid thumb deformities. *Bull Hosp Joint Dis* 1968;29:119–137
(Initally 4 types but now updated to 6)

Terrono A, Nalebuff EA, Phillips C. The rheumatoid thumb. In: Hunter JM, Mackin ES, Callahan AD, eds. *Rehabilitation of the Hand: Surgery and Therapy*. St Louis, MO: CV Mosby;1995:1329–1343

I   Boutonniere (MCPJ flexion)
II   Adducted boutonniere
III   Adducted Swan Neck (Z thumb)
IV   Gamekeeper's thumb (Subluxed CMCJ + Attenuation/ rupture UCL)
V   Isolated Swan Neck
VI   Arthritis Mutilans

**2.20.14 Harrison's Classification of MCPJ Involvement
in Rheumatoid Arthritis**
Harrison DH, Harrison SH, Smith P. Re-alignment procedure for ulnar drift of the metacarpophalangeal joint in rheumatoid arthritis. *Hand* 1979;11(2):163–168

Grade 1   Extensor tendon dislocated, No medial shift
Grade 2   Ulnar drift, Medial shift
Grade 3   Ulnar drift, Medial shift, MCPJ subluxation
Grade 4   Ulnar drift, Medial shift, MCPJ subluxation, Limited passive extension

**2.20.15 Rheumatoid Arthritis: Wrightington
Wrist Classification**
Hodgson et al. *JHS* 1989;14B:451

Grade 1   Wrist architecture preserved
          Scaphoid: mild rotatory instability
          Periarticular osteoporosis, erosions, cysts
Grade 2   Radio-scaphoid, Intercarpal joint preservation
          Ulnar translocation
          Volar intercalated segment instability
          Scaphoid: flexed
          Degenerate radio-lunate joint
Grade 3   Radius pseudocysts otherwise preserved

Degenerate intercarpal joints
Radio-scaphoid joint erosion
Carpus subluxed in volar direction on radius
Grade 4   Radius: – loss of bone stock
                  – medial erosion

Psoriatic arthritis:
– A seronegative arthropathy in which the inflammatory process involves joint synovitis, fibrosis and osteolysis. A typical skin rash and nail changes are associated. Rheumatoid factor and nodules are absent. The DIPJ may be involved which is another distinguishing feature from rheumatoid arthritis.

2.21 PSORIATIC ARTHRITIS CLINICAL CLASSIFICATION: WRIGHT AND MOLL

Wright V. Psoriatic arthritis. In: Kelly WN et al. *Textbook of Rheumatology*, vol. II. Philadelphia: WB Saunders; 1981

Different types: – DIPJ involvement
                 – Ankylosis (widespread)
                 – Rheumatoid arthritis picture but rheumatoid factor negative
                 – Monoarticular
                 – Ankylosing spondilitis

2.21.1 Classification of Psoriatic Arthritis: Kapasi et al

Kapasi OA, Ruby LK, Calney K. The psoriatic hand. *J Hand Surgery (Am)* 1982;7:492–497

1. Joint involvement EARLY, Skin involvement LATE, Arthritis – MILD
2. Joint involvement LATE, Skin involvement EARLY, Arthritis – SEVERE
3. Simultaneous onset Arthritis – UNPREDICTABLE

2.21.2 Classification of Psoriatic Arthritis: Nalebuff

Nalebuff EA. Surgery of psoriatic arthritis of the hand. *Hand Clin* 1996;12:603–614

Type I   Spontaneous ankylosis mainly affecting DIP and PIP joints
Type II   Bone loss
Type III   Rheumatoid arthritis like + stiffness

Gout:
- *A metabolic disorder giving rise to hyperuricaemia which clinically presents as an acute monoarticular episode of inflammation. The joint is painful, hot and swollen. The MTPJ of the big toe is most commonly affected. In addition to raised uric acid blood levels, urate crystals may be isolated from synovial fluid or tophi.*

Pseudogout:
- *Chondrocalcinosis most commonly affecting large joints giving rise to an acute and recurrent arthritis. Calcium pyrophosphate crystals may be isolated from joint fluid.*

Osteoarthritis:
- *A chronic degenerative joint disease characterized by cartilage degeneration and bone hypertrophy at the articular surface. Clinically pain, tenderness, reduced range of movement and joint deformity are evident.*

Heberden's nodes:
- *Osteophytes around the DIPJ*

Bouchard's nodes:
- *Osteophytes around the PIPJ*

2.22 CLASSIC X-RAY CHANGES OF OSTEOARTHRITIS

Narrowed joint space (due to loss of articular surface)
Subchondral sclerosis
Cyst formation
Osteophytes
Marginal bone hypertrophy

2.22.1 Classification of Osteoarthritis
Swanson et al. *JHS* 1985;10A:1013–1024

I   Joint narrowing
II   I+subchondral sclerosis, hypertrophic nodes
III   II+erosions
IV   III+cysts, deviation
V   IV+ subluxation or dislocation

2.22.2 Classifications of Thumb Base Osteoarthritis
Eaton RG, Glickel SZ. Trapeziometacarpal osteoarthritis. Staging as a rationale for treatment. *Hand Clin* 1987;3:455–471

Eaton and Littler. *JBJS* 1973;55A:1655

Stage I	Widened joint space, <1/3 subluxation
II	1/3 subluxation, <2 mm diameter fragments
III	>1/3 subluxation, >2 mm diameter fragments, joint narrowing (minor)
IV	Advanced. Major subluxation, osteophytes, sclerosis, joint narrowing

2.23   CLASSIFICATION OF TRIGGER FINGER
Quinnell. *Practitioner* 1980:224:187

I	Pain and nodularity
II	Triggering – self correctable
III	Triggering – manually correctable
IV	Irreducible

De Quervain's Disease:
– *A stenosing tenovaginitis at the radial styloid. Synovial inflammation of the first dorsal compartment through which run abductor pollicis longus and extensor pollicis brevis.*

Finkelstein test:
– *With the thumb positioned in the palm and the wrist deviated ulnarwards, pain is produced on the radial border of the wrist in de Quervain's disease.*

Tennis Elbow:
– *Lateral epicondylitis (common extensor origin)*

Golfer's Elbow:
– *Medial epicondylitis (common flexor origin)*

2.24   GENERAL CLASSIFICATION OF TUMOURS
Benign
Malignant – Primary or Secondary

2.24.1   Classification of Tumours of the Hand: Anatomical
Primary (Benign or Malignant):

Skin – SCC, BCC, MM, AK, inclusion cyst, keratoacanthoma (see classification of skin tumours)
Adnexal structures of skin – Sweat gland tumour
Fibrous tissue – Dupuytrens, dermatofibroma, DFSP, fibromatoses

Subcutaneous tissue – Lipoma, liposarcoma, lymphoma
Nerve – Neuroma, neurofibroma, Merkel cell
Vessel – Glomus tumour, haemangioma, vascular malformation, aneurysm, angiosarcoma
Muscle – Leiomyoma, leiomyosarcoma, rhabdomyosarcoma
Synovium/Tendon – Ganglion, giant cell (PVNS), nodules, synovitis
Cartilage – Enchondroma, chondrosarcoma
Bone – Osteoid osteoma, osteochondroma, osteosarcoma, simple bone cyst, aneurysmal bone cyst

Secondary (Metastases)

2.24.2 Musculoskeletal Tumour: Enneking's Staging
Enneking WF. *Musculoskeletal Surgery*. Edinburgh: Churchill Livingstone; 1983

Grade	Location	Metastases
Benign (G0) Low grade (G1) High grade (G2)	Intracompartmental (T1) Extracompartmental (T2)	None (M1) Present (M2)

2.25 DIABETIC STIFF HAND
Rosenbloom. *J Diabet Comp* 1989; 3:77

	Limitation	Clinical findings
0	None	Equivocal/unilateral
I	Mild	One or two IPJs involved or MCPJ only bilaterally
II	Moderate	Three or more IPJ or 1 digit + 1 large joint bilaterally
III	Severe	Obvious hand deformity at rest

2.26 CLASSIFICATION OF BURN CONTRACTURES OF THE HAND (SEE CHAPTER 11)
Dupuytrens disease:
– A fibromatosis which affects the palmar or digital fascia and may progress to contracture of the digit.

2.27 CLASSIFICATION OF DUPUYTREN'S CONTRACTURE
Mikkleson. *Hand* 8:265, 176

I   Contracture 0, Nodule/Band present
II Contracture 1–45° (i.e., Total contracture of all joints)

III Contracture 46–90°
IV Contracture 91–135°
V Contracture > 135°

2.28 CLASSIFICATION OF FIBROMATOSES
Allen 1977/Enziger and Weiss; 1983

Infantile

Adult 1. Superficial (fascial) (Dupuytren's Disease)
         Palmar fibromatosis
         Garrod's pads
         Plantar fibromatosis (Lederhosen's disease)
         Penile fibromatosis (Peyronie's disease)
      2. Deep
         Extra-abdominal
         Abdominal
         Intra-abdominal: pelvic, mesenteric (Gardner's syndrome)

Volkmann's contracture:
– The clinical sequelae of a compartment syndrome of the anterior forearm resulting in flexion deformities of the fingers and wrist (originally described as a complication of a supracondylar fracture of the humerus in a child)

2.29 VOLKMANN ISCHAEMIC CONTRACTURE
Tsuge K. Treatment of established Volkmann's contracture. *JBJS Am* 1975;57:925

Mild   – Usually affects FDP (middle and ring most commonly)
Moderate   – FDP, FPL, hand intrinsics, wrist flexors
Severe   – Involves remaining forearm flexors and extensors,
             median or ulnar nerve necrosis + /– Skin involvement

2.30 CLASSIFICATION OF SPASTICITY IN CEREBRAL PALSY
Braun et al. Phenol nerve block in the treatment of acquired spastic hemiplegia in the upper limb. *J Bone Joint Surg* 55A:580–585

Classified by response to stretch:
Severe   – strong reflex halting initial motion
Moderate – visible response
Minimum   – palpable response

2.30.1 Classification of Thumb Contractures in Cerebral Palsy
Grade 1 Contracture of basal joint (first dorsal interosseous and adductor)
Grade 2 + MCPJ (and FPB)
Grade 3 + IPJ (and FPL)

2.30.2 Classification of the Spastic Hand

Surgery of the spastic hand in cerebral palsy: report of the Committee on Spastic Hand Evaluation (International Federation of Societies for Surgery of the Hand).

Zancolli et al. *J Hand Surg (Am)* 1983;8(5 Pt 2):766–772.

Group 1	Full finger extension with wrist in neutral
Group 2	Full finger extension with wrist flexed
	(a) wrist extension with fingers flexed
	(b) no wrist extension with fingers flexed
Group 3	Finger extension nil with wrist flexed

2.30.3 Classification of the Pronation Deformity in Cerebral Palsy

Gschwind, Tonkin. *JHS* 1992;17B:391–395

I	Active supination beyond neutral
II	Active supination to less than or equal to neutral
III	No active supination, free passive supination
IV	No active supination, tight passive supination

Upper limb nerve compression:
– A nerve may be compressed at any site (including more than one, i.e., the double crush phenomenon) from its entry into the upper limb, along its course until it reaches its final destination.

2.31 CLASSIFICATION OF MECHANISMS OF NERVE COMPRESSION (FIG. 2.7)

Congenital anomalous structures
Anatomical
Postural
Traumatic
Inflammatory
Metabolic
Iatrogenic/postsurgery
Swellings/tumours

2.31.1 Classification for Carpal Tunnel Syndrome

Chang B and Dellon AL. Surgical management of recurrent carpal tunnel syndrome. *J Hand Surg (Br)* 1993;18(4):467–470

0	No impairment
I	Parasthesiae intermittant
II	Threshold – mild (SWM = 2.83–3.84)
III	Weak abduction
IV	Threshold severe (SWM > 3.84)
V	Parasthesiae persistent
VI	Sensory 2 PD mild (7–10 mm)

VII   Atrophy-mild
VIII Sensory 2PD severe (>10 mm)
IX   Anaesthesia
X   Atrophy

a) Median nerve

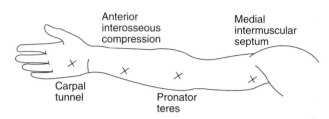

b) Ulnar nerve

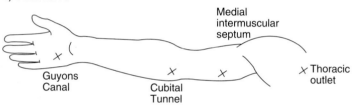

c) Radial nerve

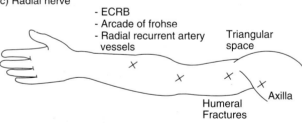

FIGURE 2.7. Common sites of compression of major nerves of the upper limb. (**a**) Median nerve. (**b**) Ulnar nerve. (**c**) Radial nerve.

2.31.2   Anatomical Classification of the Zones of Guyon's Canal

Zone 1

Area proximal to bifurcation of the ulnar nerve
Damage at this level causes motor and sensory loss in ulnar nerve distribution

Zone 2

Encompasses motor branch of ulnar nerve after bifurcation

Damage at this level causes pure motor loss to ulnar innervated muscles

Zone 3

Encompasses superficial or sensory branch of ulnar nerve after bifurcation

Damage at this level causes sensory loss to the hypothenar eminence, little and ulnar half of ring finger

2.31.3 Posterior Interosseous Nerve Palsy Classification

Hirachi et al. *JHS* 1998;23B:413

I   Complete palsy
II Loss of extension: little, ring, middle finger (recurrent branch)
III Loss of extension and abduction thumb and index extension (descending branch)

Martin-Gruber anastomosis:

– *An anomalous neural connection in which fibres usually carried in the ulnar nerve throughout its course join it from the median nerve or anterior interosseous in the forearm. In this situation, if a high median nerve injury occurs there is total motor loss in the hand, if a high ulnar nerve injury occurs there is no motor loss.*

Riche-Cannieu anastomosis:

– *An anomalous neural connection between the median and ulnar nerves in the palm.*

2.31.4 Classification of Abnormal Neural Connections: Martin-Gruber

Leibovic SJ, Hastings H. Martin-Gruber revisited. *JHS (Am)* 1992;17(1):47–53

Type I   Motor branches from median to ulnar nerve to innervate "median" muscles (60%)
Type II   Motor branches from median to ulnar nerve to innervate "ulnar" muscles (35%)
Type III Motor fibers from ulnar to median nerve to innervate "median" muscles (3%)
Type IV   Motor fibers from ulnar to median nerve to innervate "ulnar" muscles (1%)

2.32 CLASSIFICATION OF HAND INFECTIONS
O'Brien CM

(A) *Local infections of the hand:*

Digital Infection	Palmar Infection	Dorsal Infection
Herpetic whitlow	Thenar space	Dorsal subcutaneous space
Felon	Mid-palmar space	Sub extensor retinaculum
Paronychia	Hypothenar space	
(a) Acute	Horseshoe abscess	
(b) Chronic	Collar-stud abscess (web space)	
Tendon sheath		
Septic arthritis		
Osteomyelitis	Osteomyelitis	Osteomyelitis

(B) *General infections which may involve the hand:*
Cellulitis
Necrotizing fasciitis
Meningococcal septicaemia (purpura fulminans)
Others

Collar stud abscess:
– *An accumulation of pus at two or more sites between natural tissue planes which communicate with each other.*

2.32.1 Classification of Signs of a Flexor Sheath Infection
Kanavel AB. *Infections of the Hand*. Philadelphia: Lea and Febiger; 1912

1. Semiflexed finger posture
2. Localized tenderness over flexor sheath
3. Pain on passive extension
4. Fusiform swelling of whole finger

2.32.2 Microbiological Classification of Hand Infections
Bacterial
Viral
Fungal
Protozoal
Metazoal
Zoonosis

2.32.3   Anatomical Classification of Abscess Formation in the Hand

Subcuticular
Intracutaneous
Subcutaneous
Subfascial

2.32.4   Necrotizing Fasciitis Syndromes

Type I   Polymicrobial
Type II   Group A streptococcal
Type III   Gas gangrene clostridial myonecrosis

Complex regional pain syndrome:
– A variety of painful conditions following injury whereby the
  severity and duration are disproportionate to the expected
  clinical course of the inciting event. Clinically a combination of
  pain, swelling, stiffness and vasomotor changes may be
  observed.

2.33   COMPLEX REGIONAL PAIN SYNDROME CLASSIFICATION

Type 1 (Primary)   – No predisposing nerve injury (otherwise
                        referred to as RSD, algodystrophy)
                        Phases: acute, dystrophic, atrophic
Type 2 (Secondary)   – Initial identifiable nerve injury (other-
                        wise referred to as causalgia)

2.34   CLASSIFICATION OF SPLINTS

Static
Serial static
Dynamic

Chapter 3
Skin and Vascular

3.1 FITZPATRICK SKIN TYPE CLASSIFICATION

Fitzpatrick TB. The validity and practicality of sun reactive skin type I through VI. Arch Dermatol 1988;124:869–871

Skin type	Tanning response	Skin colour
I	Always burns, never tans	White, freckled
II	Burns easily, tans with difficulty	White
III	Mild burn, average tan	White to olive
IV	Rarely burns, tans easily	Brown
V	Very rarely burns, tans very easily	Dark brown
VI	Never burns, tans easily	Black

3.2 WORLD CLASSIFICATION OF SKIN TYPE

Goldman MP. Simplified facial rejuvenation.In Shiffman, Mirrafati, Lam, eds. Springer, Berlin; 2007

European/Caucasian – white
Arabian/Mediterranean/Hispanic – light brown
Asian – yellow
Indian – brown
African – black

3.3 CLASSIFICATION OF SKIN FUNCTIONS

Temperature regulation
Ultraviolet light protection
Protects against microbial invasion
Protects against water loss
Sensibility
Physical barrier to trauma
Immunological function

Mary O'Brien, *Plastic and Hand Surgery in Clinical Practice*,
DOI: 10.1007/978-1-84800-263-0_3,
© Springer-Verlag London Limited 2009

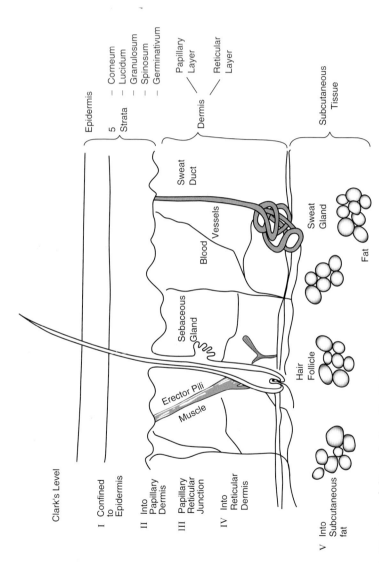

FIGURE 3.1. Structure of skin including Clark's levels.

3.4 CLASSIFICATION OF SKIN BLOOD SUPPLY

Regional deep vessels:
Arise from the aorta and form the main supply to head, neck, trunk, and limbs

Interconnecting vessels:
– Fasciocutaneous/septocutaneous (limbs)
– Musculocutaneous (trunk)

Vascular plexuses (Fig. 3.2):
– Muscle
– Subfascial
– Prefascial
– Subcutaneous: level of superficial fascia
– Subdermal
– Dermal
– Subepidermal

Angiosome
– A composite block of tissue supplied by a named source artery
  Greek derivation
  – angeion = vessel
  – somite = segment of body
  – soma = body

Choke vessels
– Reduced calibre vessels which pass between anatomical territories

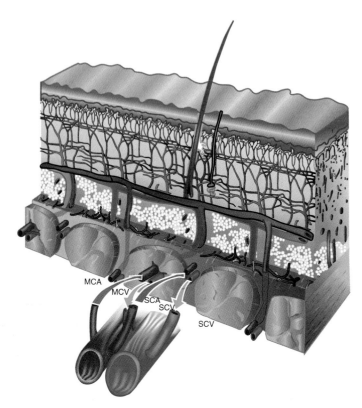

FIGURE 3.2. The cutaneous microcirculation.
(from Delaere. Laryngotracheal reconstruction. Springer, Berlin; 2004)

3.5 CLASSIFICATION OF ARTERIAL TERRITORIES

Anatomical:
– *Area in which vessel branches ramify before anastomosing with adjacent vessels*

Dynamic:
– *Area in which staining extends after IV fluoroscein administration*

Potential:
– *Area which can be included in a flap if it is delayed*

3.6   CLASSIFICATION OF SKIN LESIONS

	Non-pigmented	Pigmented
Benign	Epidermal, dermal, cyst derived	Benign melanocytic naevi
Malignant – primary	BCC, SCC, Merkel, sebaceous	Malignant melanoma
Malignant – secondary	Any source (direct or indirect spread)	

3.7   GENERAL CLASSIFICATION OF BENIGN NON-PIGMENTED SKIN LESIONS ACCORDING TO TISSUE OF ORIGIN

Epidermal origin:
Seborrhoeic keratosis (Basal cell papilloma), Actinic keratosis, Bowen's Disease, Squamous papilloma, Keratotic horn, Keratoacanthoma, Viral wart

Dermal origin:

Derivation from	
(a)	Sebaceous glands: sebaceous naevi, sebaceous adenoma, sebaceous hyperplasia
(b)	Eccrine glands: cylindroma, eccrine poroma, syringoma
(c)	Hair follicles: calcifying epithelioma of Malherbe (pilomatrixoma), tricholemmoma, trichoepithelioma, trichofolliculoma
(d)	Neural tissue: neurofibroma

Cyst origin:
Epidermoid, pilar, milia, xanthelasma

3.8   CLASSIFICATION OF TYPES OF BENIGN PIGMENTED LESION

Melanocytic naevi – Epidermal (Ephelis, Lentigo, Becker's nevus, Café au lait spot) – Dermal (Blue nevus, Mongolian blue spot, Naevi of Ota or Ito)
Naevus cell naevi Congenital (Small, Intermediate, Large, Giant > 20 cm/5% sa) Acquired (Junctional, Compound, Intradermal) Special (Spitz, Dysplastic, Halo)

Congenital melanocytic naevus (CMN):
– A naevus which presents at birth or is evident within the first 12 months of life

3.9 CLASSIFICATION OF BASAL CELL CARCINOMA (BCC)

Localized	Superficial	Infiltrative
Nodular	Superficial spreading	Morphoeic
Nodulocystic	Multifocal	
Micronodular		
Pigmented		
Ulcerative		

3.10 CLASSIFICATION OF DIAGNOSTIC CRITERIA FOR GORLIN'S SYNDROME

Adapted from Mathes. Plastic Surgery, vol. 5. Saunders, Elsevier; 2006: 399

Two major or one major + two minor required for diagnosis

Major criteria:
>2 BCCs in a person under 20 years
Jaw odontogenic keratocysts
≥3 palmar/plantar pits
Falx cerebri calcification
Bifid or fused ribs
First degree relative affected

Minor criteria:
Macrocephaly
Craniofacial abnormality: cleft lip/palate, hypertelorism, frontal bossing
Skeletal abnormality: pectus excavatum, syndactyly, Sprengel deformity
X-ray findings: vertebral anomalies, lucency hands or feet, bridging sella turcica
Ovarian fibroma
Medulloblastoma

3.11 CLASSIFICATION OF TREATMENT OPTIONS FOR NON-MELANOMA SKIN CANCER

(The appropriate treatment is patient and tumour dependent)

Surgical excision
Curettage and cautery
Mohs micrographic surgery
Cryotherapy
Radiotherapy

3.12 MALIGNANT MELANOMA CLASSIFICATIONS

Morphological
Histological: Clark's level, Breslow thickness
Clinical findings: Stage (AJCC)

Breslow thickness:
- *The thickness of the melanoma in millimetres. Measurements are taken between the overlying granular layer and the deepest tumour cell identified by means of an ocular micrometre on the microscope. It is a good indicator of prognosis in Stage I melanoma.*

Clark's level (Fig. 3.1)*:*
- *A measurement of the depth of penetration of a melanoma into the skin according to anatomic layer*

Level I	Melanoma confined to epidermis
Level II	Melanoma extends into papillary dermis
Level III	Melanoma extends to the junction of the papillary and reticular dermis
Level IV	Melanoma extends to the reticular dermis
Level V	Melanoma extends into subcutaneous fat

3.13 CLASSIFICATION OF MALIGNANT MELANOMA ACCORDING TO MORPHOLOGY

Superficial spreading	(60%)
Nodular	(30%)
Lentigo Maligna Melanoma	(7%)
Acral Lentiginous	(< 2%)
Amelanotic	(< 1%)
Desmoplastic	(< 1%)

3.14 TNM STAGING OF MELANOMA

Summarized from American Joint Committee on Cancer staging system for cutaneous melanoma (AJCC). Balch et al. J Clin Oncol 2001;19:3635

T classification:

Tis	In situ		
T1	Breslow thickness <1.0 mm	(a) No ulceration	(b) Ulceration
T2	Breslow thickness 1.01–2.0 mm	(a) No ulceration	(b) Ulceration
T3	Breslow thickness 2.01–4.0 mm	(a) No ulceration	(b) Ulceration
T4	Breslow thickness >4 mm	(a) No ulceration	(b) Ulceration

N classification:

N1	1 node	(a) Micrometastasis (pathologically detected)	(b) Macrometastasis (detected clinically)
N2	2–3 nodes	(a) Micrometastasis	(b) Macrometastasis
N3	In transit metastases/satellites or matted nodes		

M classification:

M0   No metastases
M1   Metastases   (a) Distant skin, subcutaneous, nodal
                    (b) Lung
                    (c) Other visceral/distant

Pathological Staging-Summarized from American Joint Committee on Cancer staging system for cutaneous melanoma (AJCC). Balch et al. J Clin Oncol 2001;19:3635

0	Tis	N0	M0	
IA	T1a	N0	M0	Relates to tumour size
IB	T1b/2a	N0	M0	
IIA	T2b/3a	N0	M0	
IIB	T3b/4a	N0	M0	
IIC	T4b			
IIIA	Any T,	N1a/2a	M0	Relates to nodal involvement
IIIB	Any T,	N2abc/N1ab	M0	
IIIC	Any T,	N1b/2b/3	M0	
IV	Any T or N,		M1	Relates to metastases

3.15 CLASSIFICATION OF SUNBLOCKS

Chemical (absorptive): Para-amino-benzoic acid (PABA) PABA ester Benzophenones
Physical (reflective): – Zinc oxide – Titanium oxide

3.16 WHO CLASSIFICATION OF SOFT TISSUE TUMOURS 2002

(Summary)

Benign
Intermediate (locally aggressive)
Intermediate (rarely metastasing)
Malignant

3.17 SARCOMA CLASSIFICATION SYSTEMS

(Now based on line of differentiation of tissue rather than type of tissue of origin)

Line of differentiation of tissue (tissue of origin)
Enneking
Stage
TNMG

3.18 ENNEKING CLASSIFICATION OF SARCOMA

1	Low grade	(A) Intracompartmental spread	(B) Extracompartmental spread
2	High grade	(A) Intracompartmental spread	(B) Extracompartmental spread
3	Regional or distant metastasis		

3.19 SARCOMA CLASSIFICATION BY TISSUE OF ORIGIN

Skin	– Dermatofibrosarcoma protuberans (DFSP),
	– Malignant fibrous histiocytoma (MFH),
	– Atypical fibroxanthoma (AFX)
Fat	– Liposarcoma
Fibrous tissue	– Fibrosarcoma
Muscle: – Smooth	– Leiomyosarcoma
– Striated	– Rhabdomyosarcoma
Blood vessel	– Angiosarcoma, Kaposi sarcoma
Lymph vessel	– Lymphangiosarcoma
Bone	– Osteosarcoma
Cartilage	– Chrondrosarcoma

3.20 SARCOMA CLASSIFICATION BY "TNMG" (TUMOUR, NODE, METASTASIS, GRADE)

T1 < 5 cm diameter
T2 > 5 cm diameter
T3 Invades bone, vessel, nerve
N0 No nodes
N1 Positive nodes
M0 No metastases
M1 Distant metastases
G1 Low grade
G2 Intermediate grade
G3 High grade

3.21 STAGING OF SARCOMA

1. T1or T2, *G1*
2. T1 or T2, *G2*
3. T1or T2, G3, *N1*
4. T3, *M1*

3.22 GRADE OF SOFT TISSUE TUMOUR: TROJANI SCORES FROM 2 TO 8

Trojani et al. 1984

FNCLCC system of classification for soft tissue tumours also based on Trojani (French Federation Nationale des Centres de Lutte Contre Le Cancer)

Mitotic figures (per 10 HPF) (HPF high power fields 0.1734 mm²):   1. 0–9   2. 10–19   3. >20
Tumour differentiation: 1. Sarcoma resembles normal adult mesenchyme   2. Sarcoma histological type uncertain   3. Embryonal undifferentiated sarcoma, doubtful type, synovial, osteosarcoma, PNET tumour
Tumour necrosis: 0. No necrosis: 1. <50%   2. ≥50%
Grade 1: score 2, 3   Grade 2: score 4, 5   Grade 3: score 6, 7, 8

(HPF High power fields 0.1734 mm²) Not all tumours are appropriate to grade (e.g., Well differentiated liposarcoma or Ewings)

3.23 CLASSIFICATION OF FEATURES OF A SOFT TISSUE LUMP SUGGESTIVE OF MALIGNANCY

Cardinal symptoms and signs suggesting malignancy:

Lump   >5 cm
Lump   increasing in size
Lump   deep to deep fascia
Lump   painful

3.24 CLASSIFICATION OF VASCULAR ANOMALIES

Mulliken JB, Glowacki J. Haemangiomas and vascular malformations in infants and children: A classification based on endothelial characteristics. Plast Reconstr Surg 1982;69:412

Haemangioma	Vascular malformation
	– Slow flow: capillary, lymphatic, venous – Fast flow: arterial, arteriovenous fistula, arteriovenous

3.25 INTERNATIONAL SOCIETY FOR THE STUDY OF VASCULAR ANOMALIES (ISSAV): CLASSIFICATION OF VASCULAR ANOMALIES

Tumours	Malformations
Haemangioma Haemangioendothelioma Angiosarcoma Miscellaneous	Slow Flow – Capillary – Lymphatic – Venous Fast Flow – Arterial – Combined

Vascular malformation:
- *An error of embryonic development giving rise to dysplastic vessels lined by quiescent endothelium. They are by definition present at birth and usually clinically obvious. They do not regress but often expand. They may be associated with an overgrowth of bone and soft tissue. They can be further classified as slow flow or fast flow.*

Haemangioma:
- *A vascular lesion that is not usually present at birth but occurs shortly afterward. It undergoes a rapid proliferative phase followed by involution.*

3.26 CLASSIFICATION OF CONGENITAL HAEMANGIOMA
RICH: Rapidly involuting congenital haemangioma
NICH: Non-rapidly involuting congenital haemangioma

Pyogenic granuloma:
- *A rapidly growing proliferation of vascular tissue*

Kasabach–Merritt phenomenon:
- *An invasive vascular tumour associated with platelet trapping, profound thrombocytopenia giving rise to an increased risk of intracranial, pleural-pulmonic, intraperitoneal, and gastrointestinal haemorrhage. It is associated with Kaposiform haemangioendothelioma*

3.27 CLASSIFICATION OF LYMPHATIC MALFORMATIONS

Microcystic (e.g., Lymphangioma)
Macrocystic (e.g., Cystic hygroma)
Mixed

Lymphangioma circumscriptum:
– *Small intradermal vesicles which overlie a deeper lymphatic malformation*

3.28 CLASSIFICATION OF HAEMANGIOMA RESOLUTION

(This classification is a rough guide only)

60% Resolution at age 6 years
70% Resolution at age 7 years
80% Resolution at age 8 years
90% Resolution at age 9 years

3.29 SCHOBINGER ARTERIOVENOUS MALFORMATION STAGING CLASSIFICATION

I   Blush or stain. Warm. Arteriovenous shunting by continuous doppler

II   Stage I + Enlargement. Tortuous tense veins. Pulsation. Thrill. Bruit

III   Stage I + Dystrophic changes. Ulceration. Persistent pain. Bleeding. Destruction

IV   Stage II + Cardiac failure

3.30 WANER GRADING FOR CAPILLARY MALFORMATION

Grade   I   Sparse, pale, non-confluent discoloration
        II   Denser pink, non-confluent discoloration
        III   Discrete ectatic vessels
        IV   Confluent
        V   Nodular

33.31 CLASSIFICATION OF VASCULAR MALFORMATIONS ASSOCIATED WITH OVERGROWTH SYNDROMES

Slow flow	Fast flow
Klippel–Trenaunay	Parkes–Weber
Proteus	
Maffucci	

Maffucci Syndrome:
– *A syndrome of enchondromas associated with multiple venous vascular anomalies*

Proteus Syndrome:
– *A rare condition characterized by multiple cutaneous and subcutaneous hamartomas as well as vascular malformations, naevi, lipomas, and hyperpigmentation. Partial gigantism of a limb or digit is pathognomonic.*
(The "Elephant Man" is thought to have had proteus syndrome).

Klippel–Trenaunay Syndrome:
– *A combined slow-flow vascular anomaly associated with limb hypertrophy*

Parkes–Weber Syndrome:
– *Multiple arteriovenous fistulae and usually involves a limb*

Sturge–Weber Syndrome
– *A capillary vascular malformation (port-wine stain) that lies within the distribution of the ophthalmic and maxillary branches of the trigeminal nerve. It is associated with epilepsy, glaucoma, and meningeal vascular malformations*

Osler–Weber–Rendu Syndrome (hereditary haemorrhagic telangiectasia)
– *A condition characterized by multisystem vascular dysplasia (bright red lesions) and recurrent haemorrhage. Epistaxis is the most common presentation*

Chapter 4
Craniofacial, Cleft Lip and Palate

Congenital malformation
– A structural defect at birth due to abnormal development in utero

Deformation
– A change in size or shape due to the effect of mechanical forces

Disruption
– An event that interrupts the normal sequence of development

Dysplasia
– Abnormal development or growth of tissues, organs or cells

Moss's functional matrix
– The morphology of the bony skeleton is a result of processes in the soft tissues

Frankfort horizontal plane
– A craniometric plane passing from the upper part of the external auditory meatus through the lowest point of the left orbital margin

4.1 CRANIOFACIAL ABNORMALITY CLASSIFICATION
American society of cleft lip and palate

Cleft
Synostosis (syndromal or non-syndromal)
Hypoplastic conditions
Hyperplastic and neoplastic conditions

Mary O'Brien, *Plastic and Hand Surgery in Clinical Practice,*
DOI: 10.1007/978-1-84800-263-0_4,
© Springer-Verlag London Limited 2009

4.2 FACIAL CLEFTS

4.2.1 Tessier's Classification of Facial Clefts (Fig. 4.1)

Tessier P. Anatomical classification of facial, cranio-facial and latero-facial clefts. J Maxillofac Surg 1969;4:69–92

Key landmarks – orbit, nose, mouth

0–7   Represent facial clefts (lower hemisphere) – extend down
        from orbit
8   Represents the equator
9–14   Represent cranial clefts (upper hemisphere) – extend up
        from orbit

If a malformation traverses both hemispheres a craniofacial cleft is produced that tends to follow a "time zone." The combination adds up to 14

Cleft 0   – Craniofacial dysraphia – midline upper lip and nose affected
Cleft 1   – Paramedian craniofacial dysraphia – cleft lip
Cleft 2   – Paranasal
Cleft 3   – Oro-naso-ocular involvement
Cleft 4   – Oro-ocular cleft and passes medial to infraorbital foramen
Cleft 5   – Oro-ocular cleft passes lateral to infraorbital foramen
Cleft 6   – Cleft separating zygoma from maxilla as it enters lateral 1/3
              of orbit
Cleft 7   – Cleft passes between zygoma and temporal bone
              (macrostomia, hemifacial microsomia)
Cleft 8   – Cleft passes from lateral canthus to temporal region
Cleft 9   – Lateral supraorbital clefts
Cleft 10   – Middle 1/3 supraorbital cleft
Cleft 11   – Medial supraorbital cleft
Cleft 12   – Cleft passes through frontal process of maxilla.
              Hypertelorbitism
Cleft 13   – Cleft passes medial to eyebrow. Hypertelorbitism. Widened
              cribriform plate
Cleft 14   – Midline cranial defect may give rise to encephalocoeles or
              frontonasal dysplasia
Cleft 30   – Midline lower lip and mandible

Special clefts
6   – Absent eye lashes
7   – Microtia, conductive hearing loss
8   – Absent lateral orbital rim

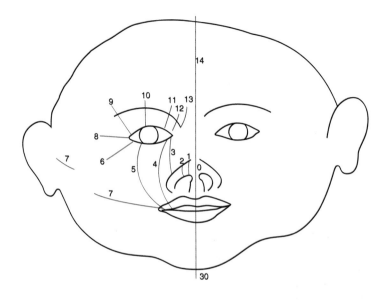

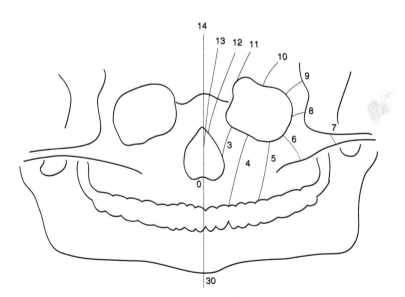

FIGURE 4.1. (**a**, **b**) Tessier's classification of facial clefts.

4.2.2 Karfik Facial Cleft Classification

Karfik V. Proposed classification of rare congenital cleft malformations in the face. Acta Chir Plast 1966;8:163–168 (summarized classification)

Group A — Rhinencephalic disorders
Group B — Branchiogenic disorders
Group C — Ophthalmo-orbital disorders
Group D — Craniocephalic disorders
Group E — Atypical facial disorders

4.2.3 Van der Meulen Classification of Craniofacial Malformations

From van der Meulen JC, Mazzola B, Stricker M, et al. Classification of craniofacial malformations. In Stricker M, van der Meulen JC, Raphael B, et al, eds. Craniofacial Malformations. Edinburgh, Churchill Livingstone, 1990:149–309.

van der Meulen JC, et al. A morphogenetic classification of craniofacial malformations. Plast Reconstr Surg 1983;71:560

Summarized:

— Cerebrocranial dysplasia
— Cerebrofacial dysplasia
— Craniofacial dysplasia:
  – with clefting
  – with dysostosis
  – with synostosis

—Craniofaciosynostosis
  – Faciosynostosis:
  – with dyostosis and synostosis
  – with dyschondrosis

—Craniofacial dysplasias with other origin:
  – Osseous
  – Cutaneous
  – Neurocutaneous
  – Neuromuscular
  – Muscular
  – Vascular

Encephalocoele
A congenital midline defect affecting the central nervous system

4.2.4   Encephalocoele Classifications

– Content of mass (Ballantyne 1904)
– Location of external mass (Davies 1959)
– Location of cranial defect (Suwanela and Suwanela 1972)

4.3   CRANIOSYNOSTOSIS

Craniosynostosis
– *The premature and abnormal fusion of one or more sutures of the skull that can appear as part of a syndrome or in isolation.*

Virchow's Law
– *Skull growth proceeds in a direction that is parallel to the affected suture.*

4.3.1   Classification of Craniosynostosis
Non-syndromic (most common)
Syndromic

4.3.2   Classification of Craniosynostosis According to Suture Affected and Resultant Head Shape

Suture affected	Head shape
Sagittal 50–58%	Scaphocephaly-keel shape
Coronal 20–29%	Plagiocephaly One fused – twisted Two fused – brachycephaly (short front to back) – compensatory turricephaly
Metopic 4–10%	Trigonocephaly – triangular
Lambdoid 2–4%	One fused – twisted Two fused – short – brachycephaly
Multiple	Clover leaf – Kleeblattschadel

Positional plagiocephaly:
– *A distortion of skull shape due to external pressure. (There is no premature fusion of the sutures and viewed from above the skull appears as a parallelogram).*

True plagiocephaly:
– *A distortion of skull shape due to premature unilateral fusion of the coronal or lambdoid sutures.*

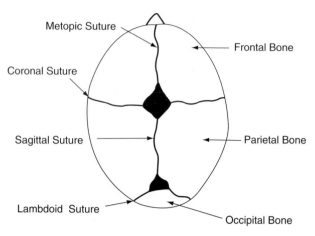

FIGURE 4.2. The bones and sutures of the skull.

4.3.3 Classification of Features Differentiating Deformational from Synostotic Frontal Plagiocephaly

Anatomic feature	Deformational	True synostosis
Skull shape from above	Rhomboid/parallelogram	Trapezoid
Ipsilateral palpebral fissure	Narrow	Wide
Ipsilateral ear	Postero-inferior	Antero-superior
Ipsilateral cheek	Backward	Forward
Nasal root	Midline	Ipsilateral
Chin deviation	Ipsilateral side	Contralateral side

Harlequin deformity:
- *An abnormally shaped orbit visible on radiograph resulting from superior displacement of the lesser wing of the sphenoid due to coronal synostosis*

Torticollis:
- *A tilt of the head toward the affected side*

4.3.4 Classification of Torticollis
Congenital
Acquired

Coloboma
- *Clefts of the eyelid presenting as a notch*

4.3.5 "TIPPS" Classification of Signs of Raised Intracranial Pressure in an Infant

O'Brien CM

T   Tense anterior and posterior fontanelles
I   Irritability
P   Papilloedema
P   Psychomotor impairment
S   Seizure, skull radiograph appearance
    (copper beaten, thumb printing)

4.3.6 Classification of Syndromal Craniosynostoses (Acrocephalosyndactyly)

- Apert's syndrome: bicoronal synostosis, midface hypoplasia associated with a complex syndactyly (see Chap. 2 for classification of hand deformities)
- Crouzon's syndrome: bicoronal synostosis, midface hypoplasia, no hand abnormality
- Carpenter's syndrome: craniosynostosis, foot polydactyly, incomplete syndactyly of hands
- Saethre-Chotzen: bicoronal synostosis, low set hairline, eyelid ptosis, incomplete syndactyly mainly second web space
- Pfeiffer syndrome: craniosynostosis, broad thumbs and great toes, incomplete syndactyly of second web space

4.3.7 Classification of Surgical Procedures for Craniosynostosis

Strip craniectomy:
- *Excision of a strip of bone over the prematurely fused suture to allow normal brain growth and expansion*

Fronto-orbital advancement:
- *Advancement of the frontal bone allowing decompression and reshaping of the cranial vault. In addition, advancement of the supraorbital bar to promote better globe protection and improved facial appearance*

Le Fort III osteotomy:
- *A midface advancement procedure by performing osteotomies to separate the cranial vault from the facial skeleton (see facial fractures)*

Skeletal distraction:
- *A midface advancement procedure involving application of a distraction device after performing osteomies*

Monobloc advancement:
- *Simultaneous advancement of the forehead, orbits and midface*

4.3.8 Classification of General Management Plan According to Age in Craniofacial Abnormalities (Multidisciplinary Team)

Infancy – Assess for: *Airway obstruction, feeding, hearing, parental support* Soft tissue correction (skin tags, macrostomia, VII graft to prevent muscle atrophy) Bony surgery: if severe (e.g., fronto-orbital advancement in craniosynostosis)
Mixed dentition: Monitor growth and development Orthodontic treatment, hearing and speech, cranial nerve function, promote maxillary and mandibular growth
Adult: Bony: orthognathic surgery, correct dystopia, bone graft facial skeleton Soft tissue augment: definitive auricle, rhinoplasty Genetic counselling

Beckwith-Wiedemann syndrome:
– *Metopic synostosis associated with a large body size and visceromegaly. May have prognathism and macroglossia. Complicated by Wilm's Tumour (or other malignancies), hypoglycaemia, seizures, and aspiration pneumonia*

4.4 HYPOPLASTIC CONDITIONS

4.4.1 Hemifacial Microsomia
Vento AR, La Brie RA, Mulliken JB. The O.M.E.N.S. classification of hemifacial microsomia. Cleft Palate Craniofac J 1991;28:68
  Grade 1–3 for each
  The acronym denotes each of the five areas of involvement:

Orbit
Mandible
Ear
Nerve-VII
Soft tissue

Orbit	O0 Normal orbit size and position
	O1 Abnormal size
	O2 Abnormal position
	O3 Abnormal size and position

Mandible	M0 Normal mandible
	M1 Small mandible and glenoid fossa
	M2 Short abnormally shaped mandibular ramus
	M2a Acceptably positioned glenoid
	M2b Medially displaced TMJ
	M3 Absent ramus, glenoid fossa, TMJ
Ear	E0 Normal
	E1 Mild hypoplasia and cupping
	E2 Absent external auditory canal
	E3 Malpositioned lobule, absent auricle
Nerve	N0 No VII involvement
	N1 Upper VII involvement
	N2 Lower VII involvement
	N3 All branches affected
Soft tissue	S0 No soft tissue deformity
	S1 Mild tissue deformity
	S2 Moderate tissue deformity
	S3 Severe subcutaneous and muscular deficiency

Associated with – Ear tags (40%), Macrostomia (60%)

4.4.2 Classification and Treatment of Hemifacial Microsomia
Munro IR, Lauritzen CG. In: Caronni EP, ed. Craniofacial Surgery. Boston: Little, Brown; 1985:391–400

IA	Craniofacial skeleton: Mildly hypoplastic; Occlusal plane: horizontal
IB	Craniofacial skeleton: Mildly hypoplastic; Occlusal plane: canted
II	Absent condyle and part of affected ramus
III	Absent condyle and part of affected ramus, zygomatic arch and glenoid fossa
IV	Zygoma: Hypoplastic; Lateral orbital wall: medial and posterior displacement
V	Orbit: inferior displacement and decreased volume

4.4.3 Classification of Unilateral Craniofacial Microsomia
Harvold, Vargervik, Chierici

IA	Unilateral facial underdevelopment
	No microphthalmos or dermoids
	+/– Vertebral, Heart, Kidney abnormalities
IB	Above + microphthalmos
IC	Bilateral asymmetric (one side worse than the other)
ID	Complex
II	Limb deficiency type (unilateral or bilateral +/– ocular deformity)

III   Frontonasal type
IV   Goldenhar type associated with upper dermoids +/–
       upper lid coloboma
       A – Unilateral B – Bilateral

4.4.4 Pruzansky's Classification of Mandibular Deformity 1969
Modified by Mulliken and Kaban in 1987

Type I   Condyle/ramus small, morphology maintained
Type II A   Condyle/ramus morphology abnormal. Glenoid fossa
             position maintained
Type II B   Ramus/condyle: hypoplastic, malformed, displaced
Type III   Ramus absent. No TMJ

Treacher Collin's Syndrome (Franceschetti: Klein, Mandibulofacial dysostosis, Confluent 6,7,8 cleft):
– *A bilateral, symmetrical craniofacial disorder with an autosomal dominant pattern of inheritance. Characteristic facies include a vertically deficient lower lid, a lower eyelid coloboma, downslanting palpebral fissures and hypoplastic malar eminences*

Romberg's Disease:
– *A progressive hemifacial atrophy which affects soft tissues (usually skin and subcutaneous tissue) but also potentially bone. It is unilateral in 95% of cases. A coup de sabre (a vertical depression extending from hairline to eyebrow) is a clinical sign of the disease*

Binder's Syndrome:
– *Maxillonasal dysostosis characteristic features include mid-face hypoplasia, a short flat nose, wide shallow philtrum and convex upper lip. May be associated with vertebral abnormalities (50%)*

4.5 HYPERPLASTIC CONDITIONS

Fibrous dysplasia:
– *A developmental derangement of bone that results from abnormal proliferation of mesenchyme. Although a benign disorder of bone that affects the axial skeleton as well as the craniofacial skeleton it may behave aggressively in the latter*

4.5.1 Classification of Fibrous Dysplasia

(A) Monostotic (B) Polyostotic

Albright Syndrome:
– *A combination of polyostotic fibrous dysplasia, café au lait spots, endocrine and extraskeletal abnormalities*

Cherubism (Described by Jones 1933):
– *A hereditary form of fibrous dysplasia affecting the maxilla and mandible*

4.6 OTHER CRANIOFACIAL SYNDROMES
Moebius Syndrome:

"Classic" definition
– *A paralysis of the sixth and seventh cranial nerves resulting in a mask like face with an inability to laterally deviate the eyes (A broader definition includes malfunction of additional cranial nerves most commonly III, IX, X, XII)*

Goldenhar's Syndrome:
– *A congenital abnormality consisting of hemifacial microsomia, epibulbar dermoids and vertebral anomalies*

4.6.1 Neurofibromatosis (NF): Classification of Diagnostic Criteria
1987 National Institutes of Health Consensus Conference

Type I (two or more of the following)	Type II
Café- au-lait spots	Bilateral VIII nerve tumours
Two neurofibromata or one plexiform neurofibroma	Affected first degree relative (NF II)+
Axillary/Inguinal freckling	1. Unilateral VIII nerve tumour
Optic glioma	2. Two or more
Two or more Lisch nodules (Iris hamartoma)	Neurofibroma Meningioma
Distinct osseous lesion	Glioma
Affected first degree relative (with NF I)	Schwannoma Lenticular opacity

Congenital dermoid cyst:
– *Benign cysts that are formed due to retention of dermal and epidermal cells into embryonic fusion lines of development. Often present in the upper lateral orbit or nasal midline. They may extend intracranially*

4.7 CLEFTS OF THE LIP AND PALATE

4.7.I Anatomical Classification of Clefts of the Lip and Palate

Clefts may be of the Primary or Secondary palate

Primary palate (cleft lip, prepalatal):
– *Structures of the primary palate are those anterior to the incisive foramen. They include the lip and alveolus. The nasal tip cartilages and floor of the nose may also be involved*

Secondary palate (cleft palate, palatal):
– *Structures of the secondary palate are those behind the incisive foramen. They include the hard palate, soft palate, and uvula*

The incisive foramen:
– *This occurs where the lateral maxillary bones meet the premaxilla in the midline and is just behind the upper front incisors*

4.7.2 Striped Y Classification

Kernahan DA. The striped Y: a symbolic classification for cleft lip and palate. Plast Reconstr Surg 1971;47:469–470

This has been modified by Millard and Jackson and Noordhoff (Fig. 4.3)

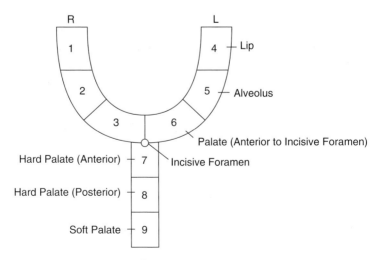

FIGURE 4.3. "Kernahan's Y".

This system diagrammatically attempts to describe a cleft of the lip and or palate. A "Y" shape is used to represent different parts of the lip and palate which is divided into numbered regions
Stippled box = Cleft in that area
Cross hatched box = Submucous cleft

4.7.3 Cleft Lip Descriptive Classification
Complete, Incomplete, Microform
Unilateral, Bilateral
Left, Right

Microform cleft (forme fruste):
– *A microform cleft is characterized by a vertical furrow or scar across the upper lip. It may be accompanied by a notch in the vermilion, an abnormal white roll and a mild degree of shortening of the lip*

Simonart's Band:
– *A band of lip tissue bridging a cleft of the primary palate*

4.7.4 Maxillary Segment Position (Fig. 4.4)
Unilateral complete clefts may be classified according to the position of the maxillary segment:

A. Narrow/no collapse
B. Narrow/collapse
C. Wide/no collapse
D. Wide/collapse

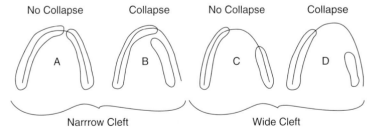

FIGURE 4.4. Classification of maxillary segment position.

4.7.5 "LAHSAL" Classification
Used by the National database on clefts

L = Complete cleft of Lip   l = Incomplete cleft of Lip
A = Complete cleft of Alveolus   a = Incomplete cleft of alveolus
H = Complete cleft of Hard palate   h = Incomplete cleft of hard palate
S = Complete cleft of Soft palate   s = Incomplete cleft of soft palate

Anatomically describes right to left
Capital letter = complete cleft, lower case letter = incomplete cleft

4.7.6 Classification of Treatment Principles in Cleft Lip Repair
1. Lengthening of the lip
2. Detachment of abnormal muscle insertions
3. Reconstruction of lip musculature
4. Accurate apposition of skin and vermilion

4.7.7 Classification of Types of Cleft Lip Repair
1. Straight line repair (e.g., Rose-Thompson)
2. Upper lip Z-Plasty (e.g., Millard) (Fig. 4.5)
3. Lower lip Z-Plasty (e.g., Le Mesurier)
4. Combination of upper and lower lip Z-plasties (e.g., Trauner, Skoog)

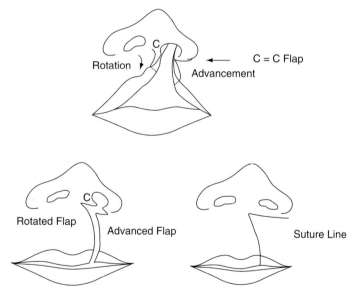

FIGURE 4.5. Millard's rotation advancement technique of cleft lip repair.

4.7.8 Classification of Timings of Cleft Lip Repair
– Traditional "10s": 10 lbs, 10 weeks, 10 g dl^{-1} haemoglobin
– Neonatal < 48 h
– Conventional: 3/12-lip and anterior palate, 6/12 remaining hard and soft palate
– Other regimes: Delaire – 6–9/12 – lip and soft palate, 12–18/12 remaining hard palate

– Schweckendick:
– 1 year lip and soft palate
– 8 years remaining hard palate

4.7.9 Cleft Palate Classification
Complete or Incomplete
Unilateral or Bilateral
Submucous

Cleft palate:
– *Failure of lateral palatal shelves to fuse with each other*

Submucous cleft palate:
– *A deformity characterized by a bifid uvula, palpable notch of the posterior hard palate and a zona pellucida*

Zona pellucida:
– *A thin, blue coloured central area at the site of velar muscle diastasis*

Pierre Robin sequence:
– *A sequence of events initiated by a congenitally small jaw that gives rise to limited tongue descent, prevention of upward palatal shelf rotation and fusion therefore resulting in a wide "U" shaped cleft of the palate*

Syndrome:
– *A collection of congenital abnormalities giving rise to a particular phenotype*

4.7.10 Classification of Syndromes Associated with Cleft Palate
Aperts
Crouzons
Downs
Sticklers
Treacher Collins
Velocardiofacial

4.7.11 Veau Classification of Clefts
Veau V. Division Palatine. Paris: Masson; 1931

Group 1	Cleft of soft palate only
Group 2	Cleft of soft palate and hard palate
Group 3	Unilateral cleft of lip and palate
Group 4	Bilateral cleft lip and palate

4.7.12 Classification of Bone Graft Timing for Cleft Palate
Primary: at the time of primary repair
Delayed
Secondary: 8–10 years, timing just prior to eruption of permanent canine tooth
Late secondary

4.7.13 Classification of Cleft Nose Deformity
a) Unilateral

Mild	– Alar base wide, Dome projection normal
Moderate	– Alar base wide, Dome depressed (minimal alar hypoplasia)
Severe	– Alar base wide, Dome retroposed (alar hypoplasia)

b) Bilateral   – Short columella, broad depressed nasal tip

Velopharyngeal incompetence (VPI):
– *Failure of closure of the velopharyngeal sphincter resulting in abnormal coupling of the nasal and oral cavities. It may result in hypernasality, nasal emission, lack of voice projection and articulation*

4.7.14 Classification of Techniques to Correct VPI

Pharyngoplasty:
– Posterior wall procedures: augmentation, superiorly based flap, inferiorly based flap
– Lateral wall procedures: Hynes, Orticochoea, Jackson's modification of Ortichocoea

Palate lengthening:
– Push-back procedures (Veau–Wardill–Kilner)

Furlow's palatoplasty:
– Double opposing Z plasty palatoplasty

Intravelar veloplasty
– *A technique to improve palatal movement*

Traffic light system for speech:
– *An evaluation system of speech represented by a visual color scheme of red, yellow, and green*

GOSLON yardstick ("Great Ormond Street, London and Oslo"):
– *A tool to assess dental arch relationships, quality of facial growth and allow comparison*

Chapter 5
Head and Neck

5.1 CLASSIFICATION OF NECK DISSECTION

Robbins KT, Medina JE, Wolf GT et al: Standardising neck dissection terminology. Arch Otolaryngol Head Neck Surg 1991;117:601–605

5.1.1 Comprehensive Neck Dissection

– Removes the contents of all five levels of the neck

(a) Radical neck dissection: – Removes the contents of all five neck levels
+
Internal jugular vein (IJV)
Sternocleidomastoid muscle (SCM)
Accessory nerve (AN)

(b) Modified radical neck dissection (MRND):

– Removes the contents of all five levels but preserves one or more of the three structures above

Medina-Classification of MRND:

Type 1: Accessory nerve preserved
Type 2: Accessory nerve and SCM preserved
Type 3: Accessory nerve, SCM, IJV preserved

(To avoid confusion it is now preferable to state which structures are spared or sacrificed as different classifications systems are not consistent with regard to structure and category type)

(c) Extended radical: Removes all five levels of the neck but may also include paratracheal nodes, mediastinal nodes and the parotid gland

5.1.2 Selective Neck Dissection

– Clears the nodes from some but not all levels of the neck due to a predilection of certain tumours for certain levels hence avoiding morbidity:

Mary O'Brien, *Plastic and Hand Surgery in Clinical Practice*,
DOI: 10.1007/978-1-84800-263-0_5,
© Springer-Verlag London Limited 2009

(a) Supraomohyoid (Levels 1–3)
(b) Anterolateral (Levels 2–4)
(c) Anterior (Levels 2–4 + tracheo-oesophageal nodes)
(d) Posterior (Levels 2–5)

5.1.3 Classification of Neck Dissection Incisions (Fig. 5.1)
(A balance between exposure and flap blood supply)

Y-shape (Crile, Conley) ("S"-shape lower limb to avoid contracture)
Double Y (Hayes Martin)

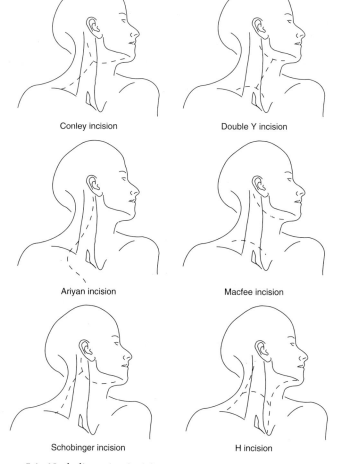

Conley incision

Double Y incision

Ariyan incision

Macfee incision

Schobinger incision

H incision

FIGURE 5.1. Neck dissection incisions.

J or hockey stick (Ariyan)
Bipedicled (MacFee) (good blood supply, consider if post DXT)
Schobinger
H
Apron

5.1.4 Classification of Defects of the Head and Neck
Hanna:
A. Mandatory
B. Functional
C. Cosmetic

5.1.5 Classification of Levels of the Neck (Fig. 5.2)

I. Submandibular triangle
– Inferior border of mandible and above both bellies of digastric
   (submandibular gland is included in the Level I dissection
   specimen)
Contents: Submental and submandibular lymph nodes

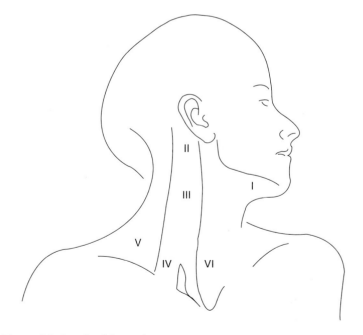

FIGURE 5.2. Levels of the neck.

II. Upper jugular
– Horizontal border: Lateral sternohyoid border to posterior SCM border
– Vertical border: Skull base to carotid bifurcation
– Clinical landmark (lower border) is the hyoid
Contents: Upper jugular and jugulodigastric lymph nodes

III. Middle jugular
– Horizontal border: Lateral sternohyoid border to posterior SCM border
– Vertical border: Bifurcation of carotid to omohyoid
– Clinical landmark (lower border) is the cricothyroid membrane
Contents: Middle jugular lymph nodes

IV. Lower jugular
– Horizontal border: Lateral sternohyoid border to posterior SCM border
– Vertical border: Omohyoid to clavicle
Contents: Lower jugular lymph nodes and thoracic duct on left

V. Posterior triangle
– Posterior SCM border, anterior border of trapezius, clavicle
Contents: Cervical plexus branches, transverse cervical artery

VI. Anterior compartment
– Vertical border is from hyoid to suprasternal notch
– Lateral boundary is medial border of carotid sheath
Contents: Lymph nodes around midline visceral structures (paratracheal, perithyroid, lymph nodes along recurrent laryngeal nerves)

5.2 GENERAL SCHEME FOR CLASSIFICATION OF TUMOURS OF THE HEAD AND NECK IN ADULTS

5.2.1 Histological Classification
Benign
Malignant
Primary
Secondary

5.2.2 Anatomical Classification
Scalp
Ear
Orbit
Nasal cavity and paranasal sinuses
Lip/oral cavity/oropharynx
Mandible, maxilla
Soft tissue head and neck sarcomas

5.3 CLASSIFICATION OF HEAD AND NECK TUMOURS IN CHILDREN

Benign
Inflammatory mass:
– Lymph node, abscess, pyogenic granuloma, sialadenitis

Tumour:
– Vascular anomaly, cystic hygroma, dermoid cyst, branchial cleft anomalies, neurofibroma, thyroglossal duct remnant, lipomatosis, fibromatoses, adnexal tumour, odontogenic tumour, osteogenic tumour, teratoma

Malignant

(a) Primary:
  – Neuroblastoma, sarcomas of soft tissue, bone tumour, retinoblastoma, salivary gland tumour, nasopharyngeal carcinoma, thyroid cancer
(b) Secondary

5.4 TUMOUR, NODE, METASTASIS (TNM) CLASSIFICATION OF HEAD AND NECK CANCER

Tumour
(T varies according to tumour site)

Oral/oropharyngeal cancer
T1 < 2cm, T2 2–4 cm, T3 > 4 cm, T4 into local tissue

Nasopharyngeal cancer
T1 one subsite, T2 > one subsite, T3 beyond nasal cavity, T4 skull

Hypopharyngeal cancer
T1 one subsite, T2 > one subsite unfixed, T3 larynx, T4 neck

Maxillary sinus cancer
T1 antral mucosa, T2 Below Ohngren's line, T3 Above Ohngren's line, T4 adjacent structures involved

Node
Nx – Unable to assess
N0 – None
N1 – Single, ipsilateral, < 3 cm
N2a – Single, ipsilateral 3–6 cm
N2b – Multiple, ipsilateral < 6 cm
N2c – Bilateral, contralateral 3–6 cm
N3 – > 6 cm

Metastasis
Mx – Unable to assess
M0 – None
M1 – Distant metastases

Ohngren's line
– An imaginary line between the medial canthus of the eye and angle of the mandible classifying localized tumours of the maxillary sinus into a posterosuperior and anteroinferior plane. It is of prognostic significance since tumours above the line tend to invade adjacent structures earlier and therefore have a poorer prognosis.

5.5 STAGING OF HEAD AND NECK CANCER

Stage 1   T1, N0, M0
Stage 2   T2, N0, M0
Stage 3   T3, N0, M0 or N1 with tumour T0–3
Stage 4   T4, N0/1, M0 or Any T, N2/3, M0 or Any T/N, M1

5.6 "S" CLASSIFICATION ORAL CANCER AETIOLOGY
Smoking   ⎱ Synergistic effect
Spirits (alcohol) ⎰
Spices (betel nuts)
Sharp tooth (repetitive trauma, ill fitting dentures)
Sun
Syphilis

Some premaligant conditions: leukoplakia, erythroplakia
(90% of primary oral tumours are Squamous cell)

5.7 CLASSIFICATION OF ORAL CAVITY TUMOUR APPROACHES
Transoral
Mandible sparing
Mandibulotomy
Composite resection

5.8 CLASSIFICATION OF RELATIVE INCIDENCE OF SALIVARY GLAND TUMOURS

	Major salivary gland		Minor salivary gland	
	Parotid	Submandibular	Sublingual	
Benign	80%	60%	40%	20%
Malignant (Primary)	20%	40%	60%	80%

Secondary
– Kidney, breast, lung, colon

5.9 HISTOLOGICAL CLASSIFICATION OF SALIVARY GLAND TUMOURS

Benign
(a) Epithelial
Pleomorphic adenoma, monomorphic adenoma, Warthin's tumour, oncocytoma

(b) Nonepithelial
Haemangioma

Malignant
(a) Epithelial
Mucoepidermoid carcinoma, adenoid cystic, acinic cell, mixed tumour, squamous cell, adenocarcinoma, oncocytic carcinoma

(b) Nonepithelial
Lymphoma

Secondary tumours
– Kidney, breast, lung, colon

5.10 FACIAL PALSY

5.10.1 Classification of the Aetiology of Facial Palsy
Congenital, e.g. Mobius, Goldenhar
Acquired (pathology at any point along the course of the facial nerve, apply surgical sieve)

5.10.2 Classification of Aetiology of Facial Nerve Palsy According to Site of Lesion
Extratemporal – e.g., Trauma, tumour (parotid), iatrogenic injury
Intratemporal – e.g., Acoustic neuroma, otitis media, trauma, cholesteatoma, varicella zoster (Ramsay Hunt)
Central – e.g., Tumour, multiple sclerosis, polio
Other – Bell's palsy

Bells Palsy
– *A temporary, unilateral, idiopathic facial paralysis diagnosed by the exclusion of other known causes of facial nerve damage. It may be virally mediated*

Ramsay Hunt Syndrome
– *Facial palsy associated with a varicella zoster viral infection*

5.11 GRADING OF SEVERITY OF FACIAL PALSY

House JW, Brackmann DE. Facial nerve grading system. Otolaryngol Head Neck Surg 1985;93(2):146–147

This system assesses gross facial function in addition to motion of the forehead, eye and mouth associated with the level of effort required

I. Normal facial function all areas

II. Mild dysfunction

Gross	– Slight weakness noticeable on gross inspection
	– Slight synkinesis
	– At rest normal symmetry and tone
Motion	– Forehead: moderate to good
	– Eye: complete with effort
	– Mouth: slight asymmetry

III. Moderate dysfunction

Gross	– Obvious but not disfiguring difference between the two sides
	– Noticeable synkinesis but not severe
	– At rest: normal symmetry and tone
Motion	– Forehead: slight/moderate movement
	– Eye: complete closure with effort
	– Mouth: slightly weak with maximum effort

IV. Moderately severe dysfunction

Gross	– Obvious weakness +/– disfiguring asymmetry
	– At rest, normal symmetry and tone
Motion	– Forehead: none
	– Eye: incomplete closure
	– Mouth: Asymmetric with maximum effort

V. Severe dysfunction, no movement

Gross	– Barely perceptible motion
	– Asymmetry at rest
Motion	– Forehead: none
	– Eye: incomplete closure
	– Mouth: slight movement

VI. Total paralysis, no movement

5.11.1   Classification of Treatment Options for Facial Palsy

Conservative: Eye lubricant, taping, glasses

Medical: (BOTOX injections to normal side to promote facial symmetry, limited use targeted at specific muscles, e.g., depressor anguli oris)

Surgical:
(a) Static	Tarsorrhaphy
	Skin excision
	Ectropion correction
	Brow/face lift
	Gold weights
	Slings (fascia lata)
(b) Dynamic	
Nerve	– Repair
	– Graft
	– Transfer
	– Cross-facial nerve graft
Muscle	– Local flaps (masseter/temporalis)
	– Free flaps (gracilis/pectoralis minor/latissimus dorsi)
	+ cross facial nerve graft

5.12 EAR ABNORMALITIES

5.12.1 Ear Defect Classification

Congenital
Acquired

5.12.2 Congenital Auricular Deformity Classification: Tanzer

Tanzer RC. Reconstructive Plastic surgery. 2nd edn. Philadelphia, PA: WB Saunders; 1977

Type:	1	Anotia
	2A	Microtia PLUS External auditory meatus (EAM) atresia
	2B	Microtia MINUS External auditory meatus atresia
	3	Middle 1/3 of ear Hypoplasia
	4A	Constricted Ear
	4B	Cryptotia
	4C	Upper 1/3 of ear Hypoplasia
	5	Prominent ear

5.12.3 Meurman Classification of Auricular Anomalies

Grade I	– Small malformed ear, most components present
Grade II	– Vertical remnant of skin and cartilage, external auditory meatus atresia
Grade III	– Almost entirely absent auricle, diminutive skin and cartilage remnants, misplaced lobule

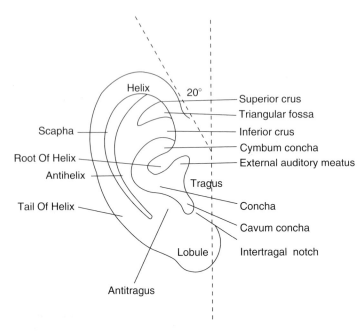

FIGURE 5.3. A normal ear showing the vertical relationship to the skull.

Anotia:
– *A complete absence of the ear. It may be associated with a syndrome such as Hemifacial microsomia (more commonly unilateral) or Treacher Collins syndrome (more commonly bilateral)*

Microtia:
– *A malformation of the external and middle ear of varying severity. The ear may range from being small to having disorganized cartilage attached to a variable amount of lobule*

Cryptotia:
– *An absence of the retroauricular sulcus causing part of the ear to appear buried*

Lop/cup ear
– *A deformity of the ear consisting of an overhang of the helix which is short, a flattened antihelix, a wide concha and compressed conchal and scaphoid fossae*

Constricted ear:
– An ear with a deficiency of the circumference

Prominent ear:
– An abnormally protruding ear with an absent antihelix, widened scaphoconchal angle, and deep concha. There is an increased distance between the helical rim and scalp.

Stahl ear deformity:
– Presence of an extra (third) crus with a flattened antihelix and malformed scaphoid fossa

Gibson principle:
– Cartilage tends to bend away from the surface on which it is scored

5.13 OCULOPLASTICS (FIG. 5.4)

Eyelid ptosis:
– An abnormal low lying upper eyelid margin with the eye in primary gaze. (The normal lid covers 1–2 mm of the upper limbus, the normal distance between mid pupil and lid margin is 5 mm)

Pseudoptosis:
– The appearance of ptosis without a true upper lid margin droop

5.13.1 Classification of Ptosis
Congenital
Acquired:
– Neurogenic
– Myogenic
– Aponeurotic
– Mechanical
– Traumatic
– Pseudoptosis

5.13.2 Classification of Factors Influencing Choice of Surgical Technique of Ptosis Correction
1. Levator function
2. Degree of ptosis
3. Level of opposite lid

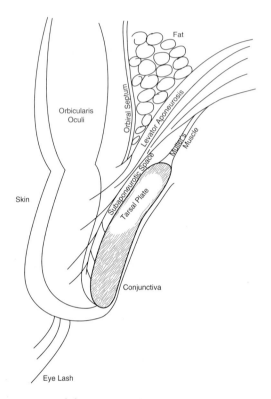

FIGURE 5.4. Upper eyelid in cross section.

5.13.3 Classification Degree of Ptosis

Mild   1–2 mm
Moderate   3 mm
Severe   4+ mm

5.13.4 Classification of Levator Function

Excellent 12–15 mm
Good   8–12 mm
Fair   5–7 mm
Poor   2–4 mm

Blepharochalasis:
– Excess eyelid skin particularly evident in older individuals

Blepharochalasis Syndrome:
– *Excess skin associated with laxity of the canthi and eyelids associated with recurrent bouts of eyelid oedema and usually presents in young to middle aged females*

Blepharophimosis:
– *Congenitally small palpebral fissures resulting from ptosis, epicanthal folds and telecanthus*

Ocular dystopia:
– *An abnormal position of the globe*

Orbital dystopia:
– *An abnormal position of the bony orbits*

5.13.5 Classification of Orbital Dystopia

Vertical:
– The bony orbital cavity is displaced up or down (not on the same horizontal plane)

Horizontal:
– The bony orbital displacement is medial (hypotelorism) or lateral (hypertelorism)

Enophthalmos:
– *Posterior displacement of the globe in the bony orbit, associated with a deepened supratarsal fold, pseudoptosis and malpositioned lateral canthus*

5.13.6 Classification of Mechanisms Giving Rise to Enophthalmos

1. Increase in orbital volume due to a blow out fracture (Orbito-zygomatic complex fracture most commonly)
2. Decrease in orbital content volume due to herniation through a fracture
3. Posterior tethering of orbital contents in the fracture line
4. Late atrophy of intraorbital fat

5.13.7 Classification of Principles of Reconstruction of Enophthalmos

Skeletal reconstruction
Soft tissue rearrangement
(Ortiz-Monasterio: Increase volume with rib;
Kawamoto: Craniofacial approach/bone graft)

Superior orbital fissure syndrome (Rochon-Duvigneaud's Syndrome):
– *Ptosis, proptosis, paralysis of III, IV, VI, anaesthesia V1*

Orbital apex syndrome:
– *Blindness + Superior fissure syndrome*

Annulus of Zinn:
– *Recti origin, fibrous thickening of perisoteum, common tendinous ring*

Marcus Gunn Pupil:
– *An afferent pupillary defect whereby light shone into the affected eye causes pupillary dilatation of the affected pupil; light shone into the unaffected eye provokes a normal pupillary consensual response (both pupils constrict)*
– *Associations: orbital fractures, globe rupture, lens dislocation, vitreous haemorrhage*

5.13.8 Classification of Anophthalmia

Primary
– Complete absence of ocular tissue within the orbit

Secondary
– Arrest of development at various stages of growth of the optic vesicle

Importance
– Development of the orbit depends on presence of a normal sized eye:
– Problems   1. Absent seeing eye
               2. Disfigurement: Orbit, lid (asymmetry and hemifacial hypoplasia)

Microphthalmia:
– *A very small rudimentary globe within the orbital soft tissue*

Epicanthic fold:
– *A fold of skin overhanging the medial canthus*

Dacrocystitis:
– *Infection of the lacrimal sac which may be congenital, acute or chronic*

Exophthalmos:
– *Excess orbital contents within a normal bony orbit*

Exorbitism:
– *Normal orbital contents within a reduced orbital volume*

Malignant exorbitism:
– *Intraorbital swelling, conjunctivitis, inability to close the eyelids*

5.13.9   Classification of the Aetiology of Exorbitism
Congenital:
– Skeletal (fibrous dysplasia, craniofacial abnormalities – e.g., Crouzons)

Acquired:
– Trauma (bony fragment), Tumour (osteoma, meningioma, mucocoele)

5.13.10   Classification of Eyelid Malposition
Jelks GW, Smith BC. Reconstruction of the eyelids and associated structures. In McCarthy JG, ed. Plastic Surgery. Philadelphia WB Saunders; 1990:1671

Entropion: cicatricial, involutional
Ectropion: cicatricial, involutional

5.13.11   Classification of Lower Lid Eversion
In Plastic Surgery. Ed. Mathes, Philadelphia WB Saunders, Elsevier; 2006:842

I	Minimal lid margin eversion
II	Moderate lid margin eversion, scleral show
III	Lid margin eversion, lash rotation
IV	Lid margin eversion, ectropion

Ectropion:
– *Eversion of lower eyelid margin away from the globe leading to scleral show and exposure keratitis*

5.13.12   Classification Aetiology of Ectropion
Congenital: Rare vertical deficiency of the anterior lamella
Paralytic-associated with Downs, Blepharophimosis, Microphthalmia, Ichthyosis

Acquired:
Cicatricial: Deficiency of the anterior lamella
              Post trauma, burn, blepharoplasty, post surgery for
              orbital fracture, T cell lymphoma
Involutional: Laxity of lid (tarsus, canthal structures, lid retractors)
Mechanical
Paralytic

5.13.13 Classification of Ectropion Treatment Techniques

Medial laxity + Medial canthal stability   = Medial Wedge
Medial laxity + Medial canthal Instability = Medial canthopexy
Lateral laxity + Lateral canthal stability   = Kuhnt-Szymanowski
Lateral laxity + Lateral canthal Instability = Lateral canthal sling

Kuhnt-Szymanowski procedure:
– *An operation to correct ectropion involving a lateral wedge resection of the posterior lamella of the lower lid*

Canthal Sling/Canthopexy:
– *A procedure to tighten the lateral part of the lower lid by tightening the lower limb of the lateral canthal tendon and securing to the lateral orbital rim at a level equal to the upper edge of the pupil*

Lateral cantholysis:
– *Division of the lower limb of the lateral canthal tendon which enables mobilization and direct closure of defect 1/4 to 1/3 the horizontal width of the eyelid*

Entropion:
– *Inversion of eyelid which may give corneal irritation from in turned lashes*

5.13.14 Classification of Aetiology of Entropion

Congenital
Involutional
Cicatricial
Acute spastic (ocular irritation resulting in orbicularis oculi overwhelming lid retractors)
Post ptosis correction: removal of too much tarsal plate

Evisceration:
– *Removal of contents of globe leaving the sclera intact*

Enucleation:
– *Removal of the globe*

Exenteration:
– *Removal of contents of orbit and eyelids*

Schirmer's Test:
– *A test evaluating tear secretion and therefore assessing the integrity of the greater petrosal nerve*
  (A strip of filter paper (5 × 35 mm) is placed in the lower conjunctiva for 5 min < 10 mm wetting is abnormal).

Schirmer's Test 2:
– *Involves local anaesthetic administration to block reflex tear secretion in addition to above*

Hypertelorism:
– *An increase in the distance between the bony orbits*

5.13.15 Tessier's Classification of Hypertelorism
Type 1   30–34 mm interorbital distance
Type 2   35–39 mm
Type 3   > 40 mm

Hypotelorism:
– *A shorter than normal distance between the bony orbits*

Telecanthus:
– *A widened distance between the canthi*

Pseudotelecanthus:
– *An apparently widened intercanthal distance between the canthi caused by epicanthal folds or a wide nasal bridge*

5.13.16 Approach to Reconstruction of Specific Facial Defects
Classification of eyelid defects

Upper lid
Lower lid

Anterior lamella: skin, orbicularis oculi
Posterior lamella: tarsal plate, conjunctiva

Partial thickness
Full thickness

5.13.17   Classification of Eyelid Reconstructive Options

Full thickness defects	Lower lid
<1/4	Direct closure of wedge or pentagonal excision
1/4 to 1/3	Wedge/pentagon + lateral cantholysis
>1/3	*Anterior lamella:*
	Skin graft
	Flap – cheek advancement (McGregor includes Z plasty) or (Mustarde), Tripier, superiorly based cheek flap, lateral nose flap, glabella flap
	Posterior lamella:
	Septomucosal graft via lateral rhinotomy incision
	Other options: Hughes tarsoconjunctival flap

(Lower lid may be used to reconstruct the upper lid but not usually the other way around)

Full thickness defects	Upper lid
<1/4	Direct closure of wedge or pentagonal excision
<1/3	Wedge/pentagon + lateral cantholysis
>1/3	Central cutler-beard flap
	Mustarde lower lid switch + reconstruction of lower lid

See Fig. 5.5

5.13.18   Classification of Approach to Eyebrow Reconstruction
Hair bearing FTSG
Pinch grafts
Pedicled flap on superficial temporal vessels

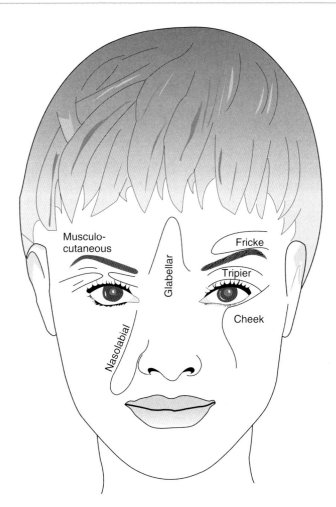

FIGURE 5.5. Local flap options for skin cover of eyelid defects.

5.14 NASAL RECONSTRUCTION

5.14.1 Classification of Type of Nasal Defect
Total: Involves part or all of the nasal bones
Subtotal: Loss of cartilaginous portion of the nose

5.14.2 Classification of Principles of Nasal Reconstruction
1. Lining: Barton's five procedures:
   • Turn in nasal flap

- Infolded extra-nasal flap
- Pre-laminated (SSG) forehead flap
- Composite nasal septal flap
- Lining advancement

2. Support:
   - Midline: L strut, hinged septal flap, septal pivot flap, cantilever bone graft
   - Lateral

3. Cover: Skin graft
   - Local flap: Banner flap, bilobed flap, Sliding dorsal flap
   - Regional flaps: Naso-labial, cheek advancement, forehead flap
   - Free: Radial forearm, auricular

(Historically tube pedicles)

Composite graft:
Provides lining, support and cover for alar defects (defect size limited to 1.5 cm)

5.15 LIP RECONSTRUCTION (FIGS. 5.6 AND 5.7)

5.15.1 Classification of Principles of Lip Reconstruction
– Align the vermilion
– Approximate the muscle to maintain oral competence

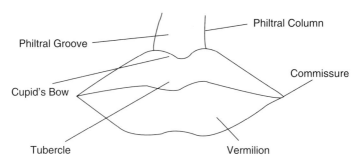

FIGURE 5.6. Anatomy of the lip.

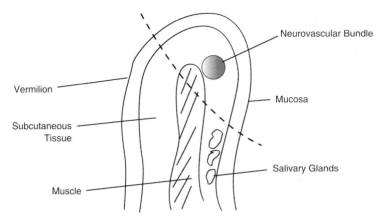

FIGURE 5.7. The lower lip in cross section illustrating the position of the neurovascular bundle.

5.15.2 Classification of Reconstructive Options for Full Thickness Lip Defects According to Size of Tissue Loss

<30%
Direct closure
(Upper lip 25% unless elderly patient with tissue laxity)

30–50%
Abbe flap (Fig. 5.8)
Estlander flap (used for commissure defects)
Johansen step advancement
Karapandzic flap

> 50%
Webster modification of Bernard flap
Gillies fan flap
McGregor flap

Mucosal defect
V–Y mucosal advancement

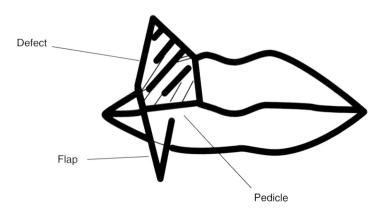

FIGURE 5.8. The Abbe flap.

5.16   CHEEK RECONSTRUCTION

5.16.1   Classification of the Cheek Aesthetic Unit and Overlapping Zones
Zone 1:   Suborbital – subdivisions A, B, C
Zone 2:   Preauricular
Zone 3:   Buccomandibular

5.16.2   Classification of Reconstructive Options for Cheek Defects
Direct closure
SSG
FTSG
Local flaps: Rhomboid, transposition
Regional flaps: – Cervicofacial inferomedially or inferolaterally based
                – Neck flap
                – Deltopectoral
                – Trapezius myocutaneous
                – Pectoralis major

Tissue expansion
Free flap – Radial forearm, TFL, Parascapular flaps

5.16.3   Classification of Layers of the Scalp
Skin
Connective tissue (fat and fibrous tissue)
Aponeurosis (Galea: a tough fibrous layer which runs from frontalis to occipitalis)
Loose areolar tissue
Pericranium

5.16.4   Classification of Scalp Reconstructive Options
Direct closure
Skin graft (onto vascularized soft tissue or after removal of outer
   table of bone)
Local flap (+/– scoring of galea)
Pericranial flap + skin graft
Tissue expansion
Free flap

5.17   MANDIBULAR DEFECT CLASSIFICATION
Bone loss is described in terms of the following:
C – Central segment, lies between the two canine teeth
L – Lateral segments (condyle not included)
H – Hemimandible segments (includes condyle)

Andy Gump deformity:
*– The deformity resulting from resection of the anterior mandible
   giving rise to loss of height, width and projection of the lower third
   of the face (Fig. 5.9)*

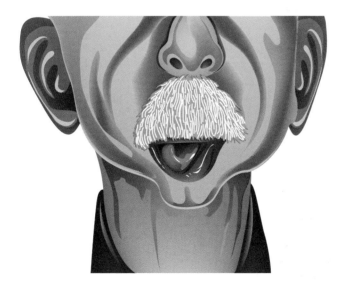

FIGURE 5.9. The Andy Gump deformity (from Laryngotracheal reconstruction,
p. 279. fig. 8.16 Delaere, Springer 2004).

5.17.1 Classification of Mandibular Reconstructive Options

Non-vascularized bone graft:

Prosthetic: Metal plates, Dacron trays packed with cancellous bone

Pedicled flaps: Trapezius, Pectoralis – osteomyocutaneous flaps

Free flaps: Fibula, Ilium, Scapula, Radius

5.17.2 Classification of Chin Deformities

Macrogenia

Microgenia

Combined

Assymetry

Pseudomacrogenia

Pseudomicrogenia

Witch's chin deformity

Witch's chin deformity:

– *Characteristic appearance of the chin resulting from soft tissue ptosis*

Chapter 6
Facial Fractures

6.1 CLASSIFICATION OF FACIAL FRACTURES
Open or closed

6.1.1 Anatomical Classification of Facial Fractures
Upper face   – Frontal bone, Frontal sinus, Supraorbital
Orbit   – Rim: Supraorbital, Zygomatic, Nasoethmoidal
             – Internal
Maxilla
Nose
Mandible

6.2 LE FORT CLASSIFICATION OF MAXILLARY FRACTURES (FIG. 6.1)
Le Fort R. Experimental study of fractures of the upper jaw: Part I and II. Rev Chir Paris 1901;23:208
    Translated by P Tessier and reprinted in Plast Reconstr Surg 1972;50:497

Le Fort R. Experimental study of fractures of the upper jaw: Part III. Rev Chir Paris 1901;23:479
    Translated by P Tessier and reprinted in Plast Reconstr Surg 1972;50:600

Le Fort I (Geurin fracture):
– *A transverse fracture line through the maxilla separating the upper mid face from the maxillary alveolus. The lower segment may be referred to as a "floating palate" and comprises of the alveolus, palate and pterygoid plates*

Mary O'Brien, *Plastic and Hand Surgery in Clinical Practice,*
DOI: 10.1007/978-1-84800-263-0_6,
© Springer-Verlag London Limited 2009

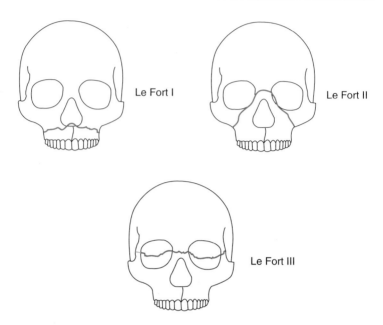

FIGURE 6.1. Le fort fracture lines.

Le Fort II (Pyramidal fracture):
– *A pyramidal shaped fracture separating the maxillary segment with accompanying dentition from the orbits and upper craniofacial skeleton*

Le Fort III (Craniofacial dysjunction):
– *Separation of the maxilla at the level of the upper part of the zygoma, orbital floor and nasoethmoid region from the remainder of the craniofacial skeleton (separation of the facial from the cranial bones)*

6.2.1 Classification of Maxillary Buttresses

Vertical buttresses:
    Nasomaxillary
    Zygomaticomaxillary
    Pterygopalatine

Horizontal buttresses:
    Frontal bar
    Infra-orbital rims
    Zygomatic arch
    Mandibular body

6.3 STRANC CLASSIFICATION OF NASAL FRACTURES

Stranc MF, Robertson GA. A classification of injuries of the nasal skeleton. Annals Plast Surg. 1978;2:468

Type I   Frontal impact, anterior part of the nasal pyramid and septum involved
Type II   More comminution of the nasal pyramid and septum
Type III   Frontal processes of maxilla involved (effectively naso-orbito-ethmoid)

6.3.1 Knight and North Classification of Zygomatic Fractures

Knight JS, North JF. The classification of malar fractures: an analysis of displacement as a guide to treatment. Br J Plast Surg 1961;13:325

Group 1   No significant displacement
      2   Isolated zygomatic arch fracture
      3   Unrotated body fracture
      4   Medially rotated body fracture
      5   Laterally rotated body fracture
      6   Complex fracture

6.4 ORBITAL FRACTURES (ALSO SEE OCULOPLASTICS SECTION IN CHAPTER 5)

Blow – out
Blow – in

Blow-out orbital fracture:
– *As a result of force to the rim or globe, pressure causes fracture of the medial wall and floor of the orbit and is often accompanied by herniation of contents (inferior rectus, inferior oblique, and fat) through a trapdoor. It may give rise to enopthalmos and diplopia*

Forced duction test:
– *A test for entrapment of orbital contents. The inferior rectus is grasped and the globe rotated in all four directions noting any restriction*

6.4.1 Classification of Surgical Approaches to the Orbital Floor

Lower lid:
      – Subciliary
      – Mid-lid
Transconjunctival
Bicoronal
Intraoral
Medial canthal

6.4.2 Classification of Frontal Sinus Fractures

- Anterior wall fracture:
  - undisplaced
  - displaced, no nasofrontal duct involvement
  - displaced, with nasofrontal duct involvement
- Anterior wall fracture displaced+posterior wall fracture minimal displacement (<thickness of the bone). Dural damage.
- Displaced fracture of anterior and posterior walls. Dural damage.+/- nasofrontal duct involvement

6.5 MANDIBULAR FRACTURES

Open (penetration of skin, tooth socket, mucosa)	Closed
Displaced	Non displaced
Complete	Incomplete
Comminuted	Non comminuted

6.5.1 Classification of Mandibular Fractures According to Dentition

Dentulous
Partially dentulous
Edentulous

6.5.2 Classification of Mandibular Fractures According to Mandibular Anatomy

Condyle/Condylar neck	36%
Ramus	3%
Coronoid	2%
Angle	20%
Body	21%
Symphysis	14%
Alveolus	3%
Midline	<1%

6.5.3 Classification of Mandibular Fracture According to Fracture Pattern

Oblique
Transverse
Comminuted
Greenstick

6.5.4 Classification of Mandibular Fractures According to Stability (Fig. 6.2)

Stable
Unstable

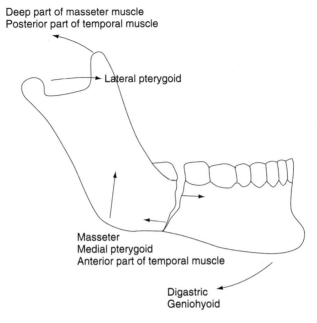

Deep part of masseter muscle
Posterior part of temporal muscle

Lateral pterygoid

Masseter
Medial pterygoid
Anterior part of temporal muscle

Digastric
Geniohyoid

FIGURE 6.2. Forces acting on the fractured mandible.

6.5.5 Kazanjian and Converse Classification of Mandibular Fractures

Class I   – Teeth on both bony fragments adjacent to fracture
Class II   – Teeth on one bony fragment adjacent to fracture
Class III   – Teeth on neither bony fragment adjacent to fracture

6.6 CLASSIFICATION OF PALATAL FRACTURES

Hendrickson M, Clark N, Manson PN et al. Palatal fractures: classification, patterns and treatment with rigid internal fixation. Plast Reconstr Surg 1998;101:319

I   Anterior and posterolateral alveolar
II   Sagittal
III   Para-sagittal
IV   Para-alveolar
V   Complex
VI   Transverse

Occlusion:
– The relationship of the upper and lower teeth

6.7   ANGLES CLASSIFICATION OF MALOCCLUSION
Edward Angle

Three classes of malocclusion based on the mesiodistal relationship of the permanent molars on eruption and locking

Class 1:   Normal molar occlusion
Class 2:   Retro occlusion or mandibular deficiency – upper molars are not in mesiobuccal groove but are anterior to it (over bite)
Class 3:   Prognathic occlusion or maxillary deficiency – the lower front teeth are more prominent than the upper front teeth (under bite)

6.8   THE "P SYSTEM" FOR EXAMINATION
   OF THE HEAD AND NECK

A systematic and comprehensive method of examination of the traumatised head and neck as illustrated in the figure below is depicted by the letter "P"

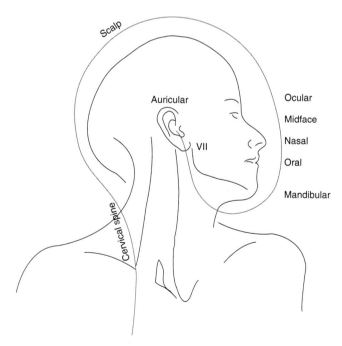

FIGURE 6.3. The "P System" for examination of the head and neck.

6.9   GLASGOW COMA SCALE

Teasdale G, Jennett B. Assessment of coma and impaired consciousness. Lancet 1974;81–84

Eye opening:
4   Spontaneous
3   To voice
2   To pain
1   None

Best verbal response:
5   Oriented
4   Confused
3   Incoherent words
2   Incomprehensible sounds
1   None

Best motor response:
6   Obeys commands
5   Localizes to pain
4   Withdraws to pain
3   Decorticate posture (flexes to pain)
2   Decerebrate posture (extends to pain)
1   None

6.9.1   Classification of Brain Injury According to Glasgow Coma Score

It is the components and not just the total score that are important when assessing brain injury

Normal	15
Mild	13 or more
Moderate	9–12
Severe	8 or less

Chapter 7
Breast

7.1 CLASSIFICATION OF CAPSULAR CONTRACTURE FOLLOWING BREAST AUGMENTATION

Baker. Aesthetic Breast Symposium. Scottsdale, Arizona; 1975

Baker DE, Schultz. The theory of natural capsular contracture around breast implants and how to prevent it. Aesthetic Plast Surg 1980;4:357

I	Natural breast appearance (Soft)
II	Minimal contracture (Palpable implant)
III	Moderate contracture (Palpable and visible implant)
IV	Severe contracture (Palpable, visible, painful implant)

7.2 MODIFIED BAKER CLASSIFICATION IN POST BREAST RECONSTRUCTION PATIENTS

Spear SL, Baker JL Jr. Classification of capsular contracture after prosthetic breast reconstruction. Plast Reconstr Surg 1995;96:1119

IA	Soft
IB	Soft but implant visible
II	Implant with mild firmness
III	Implant with moderate firmness
IV	Excessively firm and symptomatic breast

7.3 CLASSIFICATION OF APPROACH TO TREATMENT OF CAPSULAR CONTRACTURE

Capsulotomy – (closed: historically but not current practice)
           – open
Capsulectomy
Implant removal, +/– exchange

Mary O'Brien, *Plastic and Hand Surgery in Clinical Practice*,
DOI: 10.1007/978-1-84800-263-0_7,
© Springer-Verlag London Limited 2009

7.3.1 Classification of Breast Implants

Implant shape	– Round, anatomically shaped
Implant shell	– Smooth, textured
Implant content	– Liquid silicone gel, cohesive silicone gel, saline, hydrogel, trigyceride hyaluronic acid
Incision	– Inframammary, axillary, periareolar, umbilical
Position	– Subglandular, subpectoral, submuscular, dual plane

7.3.2 Tebbets "High Five" Classification

Tebbets JB, AdamsWP. Five critical decisions in breast augmentation using five measurements in 5 minutes: the high five decision support process. PRS 2005;116(7):2005–2016

1. Coverage (determines pocket location)
2. Implant volume
3. Implant dimensions, Type, Manufacturer
4. Inframammary fold location
5. Incision location

7.3.3 Scales Criteria for a Successful Implant

Scales JT. Discussion on metals and synthetic materials in relation to tissue; tissue reactions to synthetic materials. Proc R Soc Med 1953;46:647

Impervious to tissue fluid
Chemically inert
Non-irritant
Non-carcinogenic
Non-allergenic
Resistant to mechanical strain
Capable of being fabricated to the desired form

Linguini sign:
– *A sign on MRI of a linear focus of decreased intensity within a breast implant indicating a collapsed outer shell as a result of rupture*

7.4 CLASSIFICATION OF BREAST PTOSIS

Regnault P. Breast ptosis. Definition and treatment. Clin Plast Surg 1976;3:193

First degree	– Nipple is at the level of the inframammary fold
Second degree	– Nipple lies below the inframammary fold
Third degree	– Nipple is positioned at the most dependent part of the breast below the inframammary fold

See Fig. 7.1

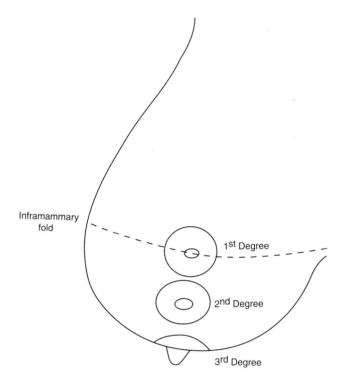

FIGURE 7.1. Regnault's classification of breast ptosis.

Pseudoptosis:
– *Majority of breast mound lies below the inframammary fold although the nipple areola complex lies at the level of or above it*

7.4.1 Brink's Classification of Breast Ptosis
Brink RR. Management of true ptosis of the breast. Plast Reconstr Surg 1993;91:657

Glandular ptosis
True ptosis
Pseudoptosis
Parenchymal maldistribution

Mastopexy:
– *A surgical procedure to lift the breast by excising skin and tightening tissues to reshape and support the new breast contour*

Breast reduction:
- *A surgical procedure to reduce breast volume and symptoms of hypertrophy whist attaining a smaller aesthetically shaped breast mound*

7.5 CLASSIFICATION OF BREAST REDUCTION TECHNIQUES

Skin pattern:

(Wise)	Keyhole
(Regnault)	B shape
(Lassus, Lejour)	Vertical scar
(Marchac)	Short lateral scars
(Benelli)	Periareolar

Pedicle:
- (Courtiss, Ribiero) Inferior
- (Pitanguy, Weiner) Superior
- (Biesenberger, Hester) Central mound
- (Orlando) Supero-medial
- (Skoog) Supero-lateral
- (Strombeck) Horizontal bipedicle
- (McKissock) Vertical bipedicle
- (Breast amputation and free nipple graft)

Closure:

7.5.1 Classification of Size of Reduction

Small to moderate	150–500 g per breast
Major	500–1,500 g per breast
Massive	>1,500 g per breast

Gynaecomastia:
- *Over development of the male breast as a result of an increase in oestrogen or decrease in testosterone or receptors*

7.6 SIMON'S CLASSIFICATION OF GYNAECOMASTIA BASED ON SURGICAL REQUIREMENT

Grade 1	– *Small* enlargement (subareolar button), no excess skin
Grade 2a	– *Moderate* enlargement, no excess skin
Grade 2b	– *Moderate* enlargement, excess skin
Grade 3	– *Marked* enlargement, excess skin

7.7 WEBSTER'S CLASSIFICATION OF GYNAECOMASTIA

Glandular

Fatty glandular

Fatty

7.8 HISTOLOGICAL CLASSIFICATION OF GYNAECOMASTIA
Florid
Fibrous
Combination

7.9 LETTERMAN SCHUSTER CLASSIFICATION OF GYNAECOMASTIA
Based on the type of surgical correction

1. Intra-areolar incision, no excess skin
2. Intra-areolar incision, mild skin redundancy, corrected with skin excision through superior periareolar scar
3. Excision of chest skin and shifting nipple

7.10 ROHRICH CLASSIFICATION OF GYNAECOMASTIA

I   Minimal hypertrophy (<250 g breast tissue) without ptosis
II   Moderate hypertrophy (250–500 g breast tissue) without ptosis
III Severe hypertrophy (>500 g breast tissue) with Grade I ptosis
IV Severe hypertrophy with Grade II or III ptosis

7.11 CLASSIFICATION OF AETIOLOGY OF GYNAECOMASTIA: 3 "PS"

Physiological: neonate, puberty, old age (increased oestrogens or decreased androgens and or receptors)

Pharmaceutical: digoxin, spironolactone, cimetidine, diazepam, oestrogens, reserpine, theophylline, marijuana, heroin

Pathological: tumour (testicular, pituitary, lung, adrenal), hypogonadism, thyroid disease, liver disease (cirrhosis), malnutrition, Klinefelters syndrome (20–60× increase in breast cancer)

7.12 TUBEROUS BREAST DEFORMITY (ALSO KNOWN AS TUBULAR/CONSTRICTED BREAST DEFORMITY)
– *A developmental disorder of the breast in which the fundamental anatomical feature is a herniation of breast tissue through a constricting fascial ring beneath the areola*

FEATURES OF A TUBEROUS BREAST
"**ABCDEF**" Classification
O'Brien CM

Areolar   – Stretched
Base   – Deficient
Complex (Nipple areola complex) – Herniated, constrictions in
                                              breast parenchyma
Difficult deformity to correct
Elongated and thin breast
Fold (Inframammary fold)   – Tight and elevated

7.12.1   Grolleau Classification of Tuberous Breast Deformity 1996
I   Hypoplasia of lower medial quadrant
II   Hypoplasia of both lower quadrants
III   Hypoplasia of all four quadrants

7.12.2   Von Heimberg Classification of Tuberous Breast Deformity 2000

Heimberg et al. The tuberous breast deformity: classification and treatment BJPS 1996;49:339–345

Heimberg et al. Refined version of the tuberous breast classification. PRS 2000;105:2269–2270

Type 1   Hypoplasia of inferior medial quadrant
Type 2   Hypoplasia of both inferior quadrants, sufficient
           subareolar skin
Type 3   Hypoplasia of both lower quadrants and subareolar skin
           · shortage
Type 4   Severely constricted breast base

Northwood index:
– *An index used to define a tuberous breast deformity*
  Ratio = nipple herniation/areola diameter

7.13   BREAST CARCINOMA: WORLD HEALTH ORGANIZATION (WHO) CLASSIFICATION

Non-invasive:
              Ductal carcinoma in situ (DCIS)
              Lobular carcinoma in situ (LCIS)
Invasive:
              Invasive ductal carcinoma (75% of invasive tumours)
              Invasive lobular carcinoma (10% of invasive tumours)
              Medullary carcinoma
              Tubular carcinoma
              Papillary carcinoma
              Mucinous carcinoma
              Adenoid cystic carcinoma

7.14 VAN NUYS PROGNOSTIC INDEX FOR DCIS

Score	1	2	3
Size	<15 mm	15–40 mm	>40 mm
Margins	>10 mm	1–9 mm	<1 mm
Pathology	Non high grade – Necrosis	Non high grade + Necrosis	High grade + Necrosis

7.15 CLASSIFICATION OF RELATIVE RISK FACTORS FOR BREAST CANCER IN WOMEN

Hulka BS, Stark AT. Breast cancer cause and prevention. Lancet 1995;197:33

Relative risk >4	Inherited mutations (BRCA 1, BRCA 2) Past medical history of breast cancer Age Family history: two or more first degree relatives with early onset breast cancer
Relative risk 2.1–4	One first degree relative with breast cancer High dose irradiation of the chest Benign breast disease: Atypical hyperplasia, nodular densities (>75% breast volume) Oophorectomy <40 years
Relative risk 1.1–2.0	Reproductive history: early menarche, late menopause, first child after age 30 years Postmenopausal obesity Has never breast fed a child Cancer of the endometrium, ovary, colon High socio-economic status

7.16 AMERICAN JOINT COMMITTEE ON CANCER (AJCC) STAGING SYSTEM INCORPORATES CLINICAL AND PATHOLOGICAL FACTORS INTO TUMOUR CLASSIFICATION

Simplified to a summary of TNM

Primary tumour (T):

Tx	Unable to assess
T0	No primary tumour evident
Tis	In situ or Pagets disease of nipple
T1	<2 cm
T2	2–5 cm
T3	>5 cm
T4	Any size, involves chest wall or skin

Regional lymph nodes (N):

Clinical classification:

Nx   Unable to assess regional nodes
N0   No regional nodes involved
N1   Ipsilateral nodes involved
N2   Ipsilateral nodes fixed to each other or another structure
N3   Ipsilateral internal mammary nodes involved

Pathological classification (beyond scope of this text)

Metastasis (M)

Mx   Unable to assess
M0   No distant metastases
M1   Distant metastases

7.17   AMERICAN COLLEGE OF RADIOLOGY BREAST IMAGING REPORTING AND DATA SYSTEM

7.17.1   "BI-RADS" Classification

0   Incomplete assessment, needs additional imaging evaluation
1   Negative, routine mammogram in 12 months
2   Benign, routine mammogram in 12 months
3   Probably benign, short interval follow-up (6 months)
4   Suspicious abnormality, consider biopsy
5   Highly suggestive of malignancy, take appropriate action

Eklund manoeuvre:

– *Displacement of a patient's implant to allow optimum mammographic screening*

7.18   STAGING OF BREAST CANCER

I, II   – Early breast cancer
III   – Locally advanced breast cancer
IV   – Metastatic disease

7.18.1   5-Year Relative Survival Rate in Breast Cancer (Classified by Stage)

0   100%
I   98%
IIA   88%
IIB   76%
IIIA   56%
IIIB   49%
IV   16%

7.19 CLASSIFICATION OF TYPES OF BREAST SURGERY FOR BREAST CANCER

Lumpectomy:
– *Removal of the breast tumour with a margin of surrounding tissue*

Quadrantectomy:
– *Removal of the breast tumour in conjunction with the entire surrounding breast quadrant*

Total (simple) mastectomy:
– *Excision of the breast including an ellipse of skin that contains the nipple–areola complex. The resultant defect may be closed primarily*

Subcutaneous mastectomy:
– *Resection of the breast through an inframammary or axillary incision leaving the skin and nipple–areola complex intact*

Skin sparing mastectomy:
– *Removal of the breast including the nipple–areola complex whilst retaining the skin*

Prophylactic mastectomy:
– *Removal of the breast prior to the development of breast cancer*
– *Three types: – Total (simple) mastectomy*
          – Subcutaneous mastectomy
          – Skin-sparing mastectomy

Modified radical mastectomy:
– *Removal of the breast, nipple–areola complex and ipsilateral axillary lymph nodes*

Radical mastectomy (Halsted procedure):
– *Removal of the breast, nipple areola complex, ipsilateral lymph nodes, pectoralis major and minor (now obsolete)*

7.19.1 Classification of Levels of Axillary Dissection (Fig. 7.2)
The levels are classified according to the relationship of the lymphatic tissue below the axillary vein to the pectoralis minor muscle

Level I	Lymphatic tissue below and lateral to Pectoralis Minor
Level II	Lymphatic tissue behind Pectoralis Minor
Level III	Lymphatic tissue above and medial to Pectoralis Minor

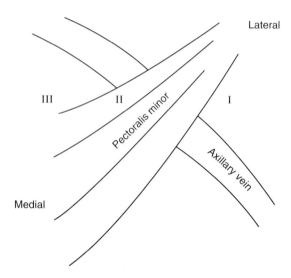

FIGURE 7.2. Levels of axillary dissection.

7.20   CLASSIFICATION OF RECONSTRUCTIVE OPTIONS FOLLOWING MASTECTOMY

Immediate
Delayed
Prosthesis
Autologous tissue: Oncoplastic or Flap (pedicled or free)
Implant/Expander
Combination

7.20.1   Classification of Factors Affecting Choice of Breast Reconstruction

Type of mastectomy
Co-morbidity
Body habitus
Smoking
Contralateral breast
Radiotherapy/Chemotherapy
Patient choice

7.20.2   Classification of Breast Deformities After Reconstruction: Mathes

In Plastic Surgery, Ed. Mathes Chapter 150, p. 1090. Saunders Elsevier; 2006

Envelope
Mound
Position
Scar
Symmetry

7.21 CLASSIFICATION OF RESPONSE TO NEOADJUVANT CHEMOTHERAPY

Singletary SE. Neoadjuvant chemotherapy in the treatment of stage II and III breast cancer. Am J Surg 2001;182:341–346

Response of tumour is compared to pre-treatment size

Complete	No measurable tumour
Partial	Greater or equal to 50% reduction
Minor	Greater or equal to 25% reduction but less than 50% reduction
No change	Less than 25% decrease or increase in tumour size
Progression	Greater than 25% increase in tumour size

Oncoplastic breast surgery:
– A combination of breast conserving therapy in conjunction with plastic surgery techniques to immediately remodel the breast following lumpectomy

7.22 CLASSIFICATION OF TYPE OF DEFORMITY FOLLOWING ONCOPLASTIC TREATMENT FOR BREAST CANCER

Clough, Thomas, Fitoussi et al. Cosmetic sequelae of conservative treatment of breast cancer. Ann Plast Surg 1998;41:471

Type I:
Overall shape of treated breast maintained
Assymetry in shape and volume when compared to contralateral side

Type II:
Obvious breast deformity
Asymmetry in volume
Correctable without resorting to mastectomy using local tissue and symmetrization of the contralateral breast

Type III:
Major breast deformity
Mastectomy and reconstruction only reasonable option to restore breast shape and contour

7.23 CLASSIFICATION OF GOALS OF NIPPLE RECONSTRUCTION

Mathes SJ, Ueno CM. Reconstruction of the nipple–areola Complex. In Plastic Surgery Ed. Mathes. Chap. 139, p. 792. Elsevier Saunders; 2006

Position
Symmetry
Colour
Size
Projection
Sensitivity

7.24 CLASSIFICATION OF TECHNIQUES OF NIPPLE–AREOLAR COMPLEX RECONSTRUCTION

Mound	Areola
Nipple sharing	Tattoo
Local flap	Full thickness skin graft

Alternatively: Prosthesis

Chapter 8
Trunk

8.1 CLASSIFICATION OF CONDITIONS THAT MAY PRESENT FOR CHEST WALL RECONSTRUCTION

Congenital: Poland's syndrome, pectus excavatum, pectus carinatum, sternal cleft, myelomeningoceles (posteriorly)

Acquired: Sternal dehiscence, trauma, tumour, infection (osteomyelitis), radiation ulcers

8.1.1 Willital's Classification of Congenital Chest Wall Deformities

Willital GH. Indication and operative technique in chest deformities. Z Kinderchir 1981;33(3):244–252

Pectus excavatum (Funnel chest) (four types) (see below)
Pectus carinatum (Pigeon chest) (four types)
Combination of pectus excavatum and carinatum (funnel and pigeon chest)
Chest wall aplasia
Cleft sternum

8.1.2 Classification of Poland Syndrome Deformities

Poland A. Deficiency of the pectoral muscles. Guys Hosp Rep 1841;6:191–193
   Clarkson later attributed the syndrome to Poland.

A. Upper limb related
   – Shortened digits (absent middle phalanx)
   – Complete simple syndactyly
   – Hand hypoplasia
   – Absent sternocostal head of the ipsilateral pectoralis major
   – Absent pectoralis minor

Mary O'Brien, *Plastic and Hand Surgery in Clinical Practice*,
DOI: 10.1007/978-1-84800-263-0_8,
© Springer-Verlag London Limited 2009

B. Other associations
  – Breast and nipple hypoplasia
  – Absent anterior axillary fold
  – Absent latissimus dorsi, deltoid, serratus anterior
  – Bony abnormalities of chest wall
  – Dextrocardia

Pectus excavatum:
 – *A congenital abnormality of the chest wall resulting in a funnel shaped chest.*
  (10× more common than pectus carinatum)

8.1.3 Classification of Pectus Excavatum
(Sub-classification from Willital's classification of congenital chest wall deformities)

I	Symmetrical depression
II	Asymmetrical depression
III	Symmetrical depression with platythorax
IV	Asymmetrical depression with platythorax

Pectus Carinatum:
 – *A congenital abnormality of the chest wall resulting in a pigeon shaped chest*

8.1.4 Classification of Sternal Clefts
Complete
Incomplete

8.1.5 Classification of Congenital Sternal Defects (Modified Ravitch)
Hersh JH et al. Sternal malformation/vascular dysplasia association. Am J Med Genet 1985;21:177

I	Cleft sternum without associated anomalies
	A Partial to complete
	B Variable median abdominal raphe
II	Cleft sternum with vascular dysplasia
III	True ectopia cordis
	A Cardiac lesions
	B Other associated midline malformations
IV	Cantrell's pentalogy

Cantrell's Pentalogy:
 – *A rare congenital abnormality characterized by defects of the lower sternum, diaphragm, pericardium, thoracoabdominal wall (omphalocele), and heart*

Sternal dehiscence:
- *Breakdown of a median sternotomy wound (in approximately 1% of cases) and is predisposed to by devascularization of sternum if one or both internal mammary arteries are harvested*

8.1.6 Classification of Infected Median Sternotomy Wounds

From Pairolero PC, Arnold PG. Chest wall tumours. Experience with 100 consecutive patients. J Thorac Cardiovasc Surg 1985;90: 367–372

Type I   – Serosanguinous discharge, no cellulitis within days
Type II   – Purulent mediastinitis+costochondritis and osteomyelitis within weeks
Type III   – Chronic wound infection+costochondritis and osteomyelitis occurs months to years later

8.1.7 The "O" Classification of Principles of Chest Wall Reconstruction

O'Brien CM

Optimize the patient
Optimize the wound (microbiology swabs and treatment, excise necrotic/nonviable tissue, vacuum therapy where appropriate)
Outline of the defect: size, location, and components
Over four contiguous rib segments involved, provide skeletal stabilization
    Autogenous tissue (e.g., rib grafts free or vascularized, fascia, muscle flap)
    Synthetic (e.g., Teflon, Prolene mesh, Gore-tex)
    Composite mesh (e.g., marlex methylmethacrylate sandwich)
Obliterate the dead space and provide cover with well vascularized tissue

8.1.8 Classification of Flap Options for Anterior Chest Wall Reconstruction

Skin flaps: Deltopectoral
Muscle or musculocutaneous flaps (preferred choice)
            Narrow defect: Advancement
            Wider defect: Pectoralis major
                           Rectus abdominus
                           Latissimus dorsi
                           Serratus anterior

Omentum (Carberry, Jurkiewicz) – for anterior chest wall or sternal dehiscence

Microvascular free flap (if regional options are unavailable or have failed) Latissimus dorsi, Tensor fascia lata

8.1.9 Classification of Flap Options for Sternal Dehiscence
Pectoralis major:
– Unilateral or bilateral muscles
– Based on thoracoacromial pedicle
– Based on internal mammary artery perforators as a turnover flap

Rectus abdominus:
– Based on the superior epigastric pedicle

8.2 Classification of Posterior Chest Wall Muscle Flap Reconstructive Options
(Defects may be congenital or acquired complications of neurosurgical or orthopaedic surgery)

Latissimus Dorsi: Advancement or turnover (based on secondary paraspinal perforators)

Trapezius: Advancement or turnover (based on secondary paraspinal perforators)

8.2.1 Congenital Abnormalities of the Abdominal Wall
Gastroschisis:
– *A congenital condition whereby the intestine and possibly other viscera herniate outside the foetal abdomen through an opening in the abdominal wall usually to the right of the umbilicus*

Omphalocele:
– *A congenital condition whereby the intestine and possibly other viscera herniate through the umbilical ring into the umbilical cord and develop outside the foetal abdomen. The intestine and viscera are surrounded by a membranous sac of amnion and parietal peritoneum rather than being in direct continuity with the amniotic cavity*

Bladder extrophy:
See Chapter 10

8.2.2 Principles of Abdominal Wall Reconstruction
Protection of intra-abdominal viscera
Repair abdominal wall support mechanism
Prevention of further herniation
Provide an acceptable contour

8.2.3   Classification of Abdominal Wall Reconstructive Options

Direct closure

Mesh

Skin graft

Local tissue techniques:
– Components separation
– Tissue expansion
– Fascial release

Pedicled flaps:
– Tensor fascia lata
– Rectus femoris
– Vastus lateralis
– Gracilis

Free tissue transfer

Component separation:
– *Mobilization and advancement of separate layers of the abdominal wall to achieve midline closure (Fig. 8.1)*

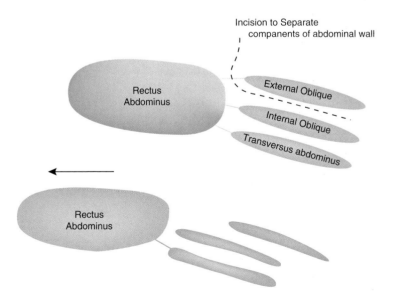

FIGURE 8.1. Components separation method of abdominal wall closure.

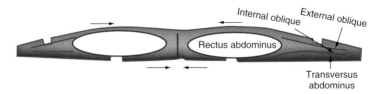

FIGURE 8.2. Fascial partition release.

Fascial partition release:
– *The use of vertical parasagittal relaxing incisions in the external oblique and transversus abdominus muscles to allow medial advancement and anterior abdominal wall defect closure (Fig. 8.2)*

8.2.4 Abdominal Reconstructive Flap Options: Classification by Location of Defect
Adapted from Plastic Surgery. Ed Mathes. Vol. 1 447 Saunders Elsevier; 2006

Zone 1 (superior half)	Rectus abdominus superiorly based or advancement
Zone 1 (inferior half)	Rectus abdominus inferiorly based or advancement, TFL, Rectus femoris
Zone 2	LD, Rectus abdominus superiorly based, TFL
Zone 3	Rectus abdominus inferiorly based, external oblique advancement, TFL, Rectus femoris

8.2.5 Abdominal Reconstructive Flap Options: Classification by Type of Flap
Adapted from Plastic Surgery. Ed Mathes. Vol. 1, 447. Saunders Elsevier; 2006

Regional	Rectus abdominus, external oblique
Distant	TFL, LD, Rectus femoris
Free tissue transfer	TFL, LD, Rectus femoris, Anterolateral thigh flap, Groin flap

8.2.6 Classification of Abdominal Visceral Flaps

Adapted from Plastic Surgery. Ed Mathes. Vol 1, 379. Elsevier Saunders; 2006

Based on the muscle classification system:

Type I	Colon, Jejunum	One vascular arcade with a single dominant vessel
Type III	Omentum	Two dominant arcades or pedicles

8.2.7 Classification of Visceral Blood Supply

Coeliac axis	– Foregut
Superior mesenteric axis	– Midgut
Inferior mesenteric axis	– Hindgut

8.3 PRESSURE SORES

Pressure sore:
- *A wound acquired from pressure over a bony prominence resulting from extrinsic factors propagated by intrinsic factors. The visible pressure sore represents the "tip of the iceberg" of a cone distribution of tissue destruction*

Decubitus ulcer derivation:
- *Decumbere (Latin) = "to lie down"*

8.3.1 Classification of Pressure Sore Pathogenesis

(a) Extrinsic factors: Pressure (>32mmHg), shear, friction

(b) Intrinsic factors:
- General: Age (old), incontinence, malnutrition (Mnemonic "AIM")
- Wound: Neuropathy (sensory/autonomic), ischaemia, fibrosis, infection

Shear:
- *A mechanical stress perpendicular to surface of skin resulting in kinked vessels and reduced perfusion*

Friction:
- *Two surfaces which move across each other causing loss of the superficial layer of epidermis*

8.3.2 Classification of Pressure Sore Risk Factors

From Waterlow J. A risk assessment card. Nurs Times 1985;81(48): 49–55

Waterlow Score summarized into "ABC'S":
- 10 at risk
- 15 high risk
- 20 very high risk

Risk scale which scores:

A – Appetite, age/sex, ambulation(mobility), anaemia
B – Build and weight
C – Continence
S – Skin type
    Steroids/NSAIDS
    Smoking
    Surgery: previous orthopaedic or fracture below waist
    Sensory disturbance: diabetes, paraplegia, CVA

8.3.3 Pressure Sore Staging Systems

8.3.4 Shea's Classification

Shea JD. Pressure sores: classification and management. Clin Orthop 1975;112:89

Grade I	Ulcer confined to epidermis and superficial dermis
Grade II	Ulcer extends through the skin into subcutaneous fat
Grade III	Ulcer extends into underlying muscle
Grade IV	Ulcer invades bone or joint

8.3.5 Barczak's Classification

Barczak et al. Adv Wound Care 1997;10(4):18–26

1 Nonblanchable erythema for >1h after relief of pressure
2 Breach in the dermis
3 Subcutaneous destruction to muscle
4 Bone/joint involvement

8.3.6 National Pressure Ulcer Advisory Panel's Classification 1989

National Pressure Ulcer Advisory Panel 1989

1. Non blanchable erythema of intact skin
2. Partial thickness loss: breach of epidermis/dermis-blistering and ulceration

3. Full thickness loss: subcutaneous involvement not breaching fascia
4. Breach in fascia: extends to bone, muscle, tendon, joint capsule, extensive destruction

8.3.7 Classification of Pressure Sores by Anatomical Frequency in Paraplegic Patients

Dansereau et al. Closure of decubiti in paraplegics. Plast Reconstr Surg 1964;33:474

Ischial	28%
Trochanteric	19%
Sacral	17%
Heel	9%
Malleolar	5%
Pretibial	5%
Patellar	4%
Other	13%

8.3.8 Classification of Pressure Sore Treatment Principles

(a) Prevention – Awareness
   – Pressure relief
   – Low air loss mattress
   – Seated patients: 10s lift every 10min
   – Bed bound: 2h repositioning
   – Skin care: clean, dry, remove particulate matter, treat infection
   – Urinary/faecal diversion
   – Nutrition

(b) Multidisciplinary care – Nursing, Occupational therapy, Dietician, Orthotics, Surgical

(c) Surgical care – Debridement: scar, bursa, bony spurs, soft tissue calcification
   – Dead space obliteration
   – Durable resurfacing
   – Judicious choice of flaps to avoid wastage
   – Careful positioning of suture lines away from pressure areas
   – Adequate drainage under flap
   – Optimize patient pre and postoperatively (Figs. 8.3, 8.4)

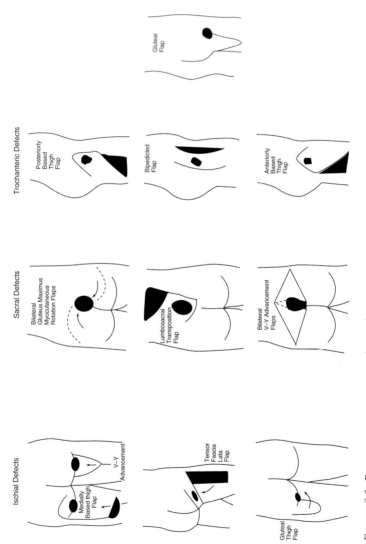

FIGURE 8.3. Pressure sore reconstructive options.

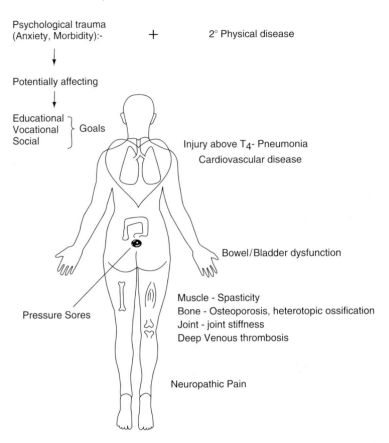

Psychological trauma
(Anxiety, Morbidity):-   +   2° Physical disease

Potentially affecting

Educational ⎤
Vocational ⎬ Goals
Social   ⎦

Injury above T₄- Pneumonia
Cardiovascular disease

Bowel/Bladder dysfunction

Pressure Sores

Muscle - Spasticity
Bone - Osteoporosis, heterotopic ossification
Joint - joint stiffness
Deep Venous thrombosis

Neuropathic Pain

FIGURE 8.4. "Top to toe" diagrammatic classification of the problems of paraplegia (O'Brien CM).

Chapter 9
Lower Limb

9.1 CLASSIFICATION OF OPEN TIBIAL FRACTURES (GUSTILLO ET AL.)

Gustillo et al. The management of open fractures. JBJS Am 1990;72:299–304

I   Bone: Simple non-comminuted fracture/Soft tissues <1 cm clean puncture

II   Bone: Moderately comminuted fracture/Soft tissues >1 cm laceration

III   High energy:
     Bone: Comminuted/segmental/bone loss/amputation
     Soft tissues: Extensive damage >10 cm long wound
     Subtype (1984):
     (a) Adequate soft tissue cover
     (b) Periosteal stripping, bone loss and exposure, major contamination
     (c) Soft tissue injury + Arterial injury requiring repair

9.2 CLASSIFICATION OF OPEN TIBIAL FRACTURES (BYRD AND SPICER)

Byrd HS, Spicer TE, Cierny G. Management of open tibial fractures. PRS 1989;76:159

Type I:
Low energy, <2 cm laceration, relatively clean wound. Fracture pattern: spiral or oblique

Mary O'Brien, *Plastic and Hand Surgery in Clinical Practice*,
DOI: 10.1007/978-1-84800-263-0_9,
© Springer-Verlag London Limited 2009

Type II:

Moderate energy >2 cm laceration, Moderate muscle and skin contusion. Fracture pattern: comminuted or displaced

Type III:

High energy, Extensive skin loss, devitalized muscle. Fracture pattern: displaced, severely comminuted, segmental

Type IV:

Extreme energy (e.g., gunshot) + crush or degloving, vascular injury requiring repair. Fracture pattern as in Type III

9.3 MANGLED EXTREMITY SEVERITY SCORE – "MESS"

Johansen K, Daines M, Howey T et al. Objective criteria accurately predict amputation following lower extremity trauma. J Trauma 1990;30:568

Score of 6 or less: Salvageable limb
Score of 7 or more: Unlikely salvage

(A) Bone/soft tissue injury:

Low energy	1
Medium energy	2
High energy	3
Very high energy	4

(B) Limb ischaemia (double if greater than 6 h)

Pulse reduced, perfusion normal	1
Pulseless, parasthetic with decreased capillary refill	2
Cool, parasthetic, insensate, numb	3

(C) Shock

Systolic >90	0
Transient hypotension	1
Persistent hypotension	2

(D) Age

<30	0
30–50	1
>50	2

9.4 HIDALGO AND SHAW CLASSIFICATION OF FOOT TRAUMA

Hidalgo DA, Shaw WW. Reconstruction of foot injuries. Clin Plast Surg 1986;13(4):663–80

Type I – Small soft tissue loss <3 cm²
Type II – Large tissue loss >3 cm² without bone involvement
Type III – Large tissue loss with bone involvement

9.5 ORTHOPAEDIC TRAUMA ASSOCIATION CLASSIFICATION OF LONG BONE FRACTURES

Linear (transverse, oblique, spiral)
Comminuted (<50%, >50%, butterfly <50%, butterfly >50%)
Segmental (two level, three level, longitudinal split, comminuted)
Bone loss (<50%, >50%, complete)

9.6 SOFT TISSUE INJURY CLASSIFICATION OVER CLOSED FRACTURES

Tscherne H, Gotzen L. Fractures with soft tissue injuries. New York: Springer; 1984

Grade 0	– Minimal damage
	– Simple fracture patterns
Grade 1	– Superficial abrasion or contusion caused by pressure from within
	– Mild-moderate fracture pattern
Grade 2	– Deep abrasion with localized muscle contusion
	– Possible compartment syndrome
Grade 3	– Extensive contusion or crush, degloving, vascular injury

9.7 CLASSIFICATION OF OPTIONS FOR MANAGING BONY DEFECTS ACCORDING TO SIZE

<6 cm bone defect: Bone graft, Ilizarov technique
>6 cm bone defect: – Pedicled bone flaps
                   – Free vascularized bone flap transfer

The Ilizarov Technique:
– A method of distraction histiogenesis (leg lengthening) comprising of the following sequence
   (1) Application of a stable external fixation device
   (2) Bony corticotomy causing minimal disruption to blood supply
   (3) Latent period
   (4) Gradual rhythmic distraction

Congenital pseudoarthrosis:
– Maldevelopment of a major bony articulation

9.8 BOYD CLASSIFICATION OF CONGENITAL PSEUDOARTHROSIS

I   Anterior bowing, present at birth
II Hourglass constriction present at birth
III Congenital cyst
IV Sclerotic segment with medullary obliteration
V   Dysplastic fibula
VI Interosseous neurofibroma or schwannoma

Acquired pseudoarthrosis:
– A chronically unstable bone union at a fracture site

Ulcer:
– A breach in the epithelium with one or more factors preventing it from healing

9.9 CLASSIFICATION OF LEG ULCER AETIOLOGY

Venous disease
Arterial disease
Trauma: direct, deliberate self-harm, bites, frostbite, radiation
Tumour: BCC, SCC (Marjolin's ulcer), lymphoma, Kaposi
Infection: bacterial, fungal, TB, Syphilis
Metabolic: pyoderma, necrobiosis lipoidica diabetorum, gout
Autoimmune: rheumatoid, polyarteritis, lupus
Neuropathic: diabetes

Marjolin's ulcer:
– The formation of carcinoma within a burn scar (as originally described) but now has a wider definition which includes malignant transformation within a chronic wound

9.10 CLASSIFICATION OF THE MECHANISMS INVOLVED IN VENOUS ULCER PRODUCTION

Venous hypertension
Valvular incompetence (secondary to thrombophlebitis)
Protein exudate accumulation in soft tissues
Lipodermatosclerosis

Osteomyelitis:
An infection of bone potentially resulting in necrosis within a compromised skin envelope

9.11 OSTEOMYELITIS CLASSIFICATION

Acute: Haematogenous or Direct spread
Subacute
Chronic

9.11.1 Classification of Osteomyelitis: Cierny and Mader

Cierny G III, Mader JT. Approach to adult osteomyelitis. Orthop Rev 1987

Anatomic criteria:
Type I   Medullary/endosteal lesion
Type II   Superficial
Type III   Localized
Type IV   Diffuse

Physiologic criteria:
Class A   Normal host response
Class B   Compromised wound healing
Class C   Potentially worsening

Compartment syndrome:
– *A clinical condition arising from an increase in intracompartmental tissue pressure which potentially compromises the circulation causing ischaemia and destroying function*
Pressures suggestive of a compartment syndrome:
– *Compartment Pressure >30 mmHg in a normotensive patient*
– *Compartment Pressure <30 mmHg below diastolic blood pressure*
  Described thresholds are guidelines only, the diagnosis is a clinical one

9.12 "P" CLASSIFICATION OF COMPARTMENT SYNDROME DIAGNOSTIC FEATURES

Pain out of proportion to injury
Pain on passive extension
Pain on palpation of the compartment
Parasthesiae
Pulselessness: occurs late, presence of a pulse does not exclude a compartment syndrome
Pressures (intracompartmental)   >30 mmHg
                                  <30 mmHg below diastolic

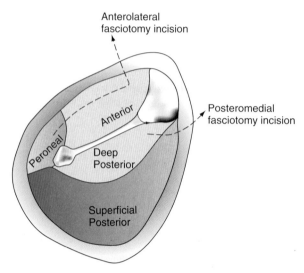

FIGURE 9.1. Decompression of the four anatomical compartments of the lower leg.

9.13 CLASSIFICATION OF TYPES OF LYMPHOEDEMA

(a) Primary (classified by age):
   Lymphoedema congenita *(20%) – Early childhood*
   Lymphoedema praecox *(70%) – Puberty*
   Lymphoedema tarda *(10%) – >35 years*

(b) Secondary:
   Trauma
   Tumour (primary/secondary)
   Infection (e.g., Wucheria bancrofti – filariasis-most common cause worldwide)
   Inflammation
   Irradiation
   Iatrogenic (e.g., Block dissection/Varicose vein stripping)

Lipoedema:
– *An abnormal collection of subcutaneous fat between the hip and the ankle, sparing the feet*

Stemmer sign:
– *Inability to tent the skin over the toes*
  – *Positive in lymphoedema*
  – *Negative in lipoedema*

Lymphoedema:
– An abnormal collection of interstitial fluid

9.13.1 Wolf and Kinmonth Classification of Primary Lymphoedema

Classified according to lymphangiography appearance

Anaplastic		Associated with lymphoedema congenita
Hypoplastic	(a) Obstructive (b) Non obstructive	Associated with lymphoedema praecox
Hyperplastic		Associated with lymphoedema tarda

9.14 COMPRESSION BANDAGES

Thomas S. Bandages and bandaging. Nurs Stand 1990;4(39 Suppl.):4–6

Light compression 14–17 mmHg at ankle
Moderate compression 18–24 mmHg at ankle
High compression 25–35 mmHg at ankle
Extra high compression 60 mmHg at ankle

9.15 BRITISH STANDARDS INSTITUTE: THREE CLASSES OF COMPRESSION STOCKINGS

Class I   14–18 mmHg
Class II   18–24 mmHg
Class III 25–35 mmHg

Ankle/Brachial index:
– A value calculated by dividing pressure measured at the ankle by brachial systolic pressure to indicate the relative degree of lower limb ischaemia

Normal index = 1.0
Index acceptable for most reconstructive techniques = 0.7
Index correlating with rest pain, nonhealing wounds = 0.3

9.16 SANTANELLI DESCRIPTIVE CLASSIFICATION OF FOOT DEFECTS

Extension
Depth
Localization
Aetiology

9.16.1 Classification of Reconstructive Options for Heel Pressure Sores

Conservative: Dressings, Vacuum therapy

Skin graft

Local flaps: – Sural artery
 – Lateral calcaneal artery
 – Medial plantar
Free tissue – Radial forearm, serratus

9.17 DIABETIC FOOT ULCER: WAGNER SCALE 1981

Wagner, The dysvascular foot; a system for diagnosis and treatment. FW Foot Ankle 1981;2:64

Grade 0 At risk foot
Grade 1 Superficial ulcer, not clinically infected
Grade 2 Deeper ulcer, often infected, no osteomyelitis
Grade 3 Deeper ulcer, abscess formation, osteomyelitis
Grade 4 Localized gangrene (toe, forefoot, heel)
Grade 5 Gangrene whole foot

9.17.1 Classification of Local Reconstructive Flap Options for the Foot

Ankle and Dorsum:
– Abductor hallucis, Abductor digiti minimi, extensor digitorum brevis, sural neurocutaneous, lateral supramalleolar

Plantar Forefoot:
– Toe fillet, neurovascular island, V-Y plantar, suprafascial

Midfoot:
– Neurovascular island, V-Y advancement, suprafascial

Hindfoot:
– Abductor hallucis, flexor digitorum brevis, abductor digiti minimi, medial plantar artery flap, sural artery flap

Chapter 10
Urogenital Tract

Hypospadias:
- *A congenital abnormality characterized by a triad of features which include an abnormally proximal urethral meatus positioned on the ventral aspect of the penis, a hooded prepuce and chordee. Associated conditions include inguinal hernia, undescended testes, paraurethral sinuses, urethral valves and a flattened glans penis, and other genito-urinary tract abnormalities*

Chordee:
- *Ventral curvature of the penis due to the presence of a fibrous band between the meatus and glans*

Horton test:
- *An artificial erection test used to assess the degree of chordee. It involves the injection of normal saline into one of the corpora cavernosa of the penis after application of a tourniquet around the base of the penis*

10.1 CLASSIFICATION OF HYPOSPADIAS ACCORDING TO POSITION OF THE MEATUS (AFTER CORRECTION OF THE ASSOCIATED CHORDEE)

Distal:

Glanular
Coronal
Subcoronal
Distal shaft
} 75%

Mary O'Brien, *Plastic and Hand Surgery in Clinical Practice*,
DOI: 10.1007/978-1-84800-263-0_10,
© Springer-Verlag London Limited 2009

Proximal:

Midshaft	15%	
Proximal shaft		
Penoscrotal		10%
Scrotal		
Perineal		

10.1.1 Classification of Corrective Techniques for Hypospadias

Urethral advancement
On lay procedures
In lay procedures
One stage
Two stage

Epispadias and Bladder extrophy:
- *A congenital abnormality of the external genitalia and bladder resulting in failure of normal development of the dorsal surface of the penis, abdomen and anterior bladder wall*

Micropenis:
- *A penis that is more than two standard deviations smaller than the norm expected for that age*

Buried penis:
- *A normal sized penis for age but hidden from view due to excessive peri-perineal fat and subcutaneous tissue*

Peyronie's disease:
- *A disease characterized by fibrous nodules within the tunica albuginea of the corpora cavernosa giving rise to a dorsal curvature of the penis. It is associated with veno-occlusive dysfunction*

Fournier's gangrene:
- *Necrotising fasciitis of the perineum and genitalia caused by a mixture of gram-positive and gram-negative organisms and anaerobes (Clostridium perfringens). Predisposing conditions include diabetes mellitus, alcoholism, smoking, leukaemia, and immunosuppression*

Balanitis xerotica obliterans:
- *A genital form of lichen sclerosis et atrophicus which may be caused by the spirochete Borrelia burgdorferi. White patches develop on the glans and can spread in a retrograde fashion along*

the urethra giving rise to stenosis of the meatus and urethral strictures. It may predispose to malignant change

10.2 CLASSIFICATION OF SYNDROMES CAUSING AMBIGUOUS GENITALIA AND ASSOCIATED CHROMOSOMAL ABNORMALITY

Syndrome	Genetics	Abnormality
Congenital adrenal hyperplasia (Female pseudohermaphroditism) (Adrenogenital syndrome)	46XX	21 hydroxylase deficiency Over exposure to androgens
Male pseudohermaphroditism	46XY	5 alpha reductase deficiency Incomplete masculinization
Mixed gonadal dysgenesis	46XY or 46XO	1 Testis/1 streak gonad (Malignant potential)
True hermaphroditism	46XX	1 Ovary/1 Testis Well differentiated male and female tissue in same individual

Vaginal agenesis (Mayer-Rokitansky-Kuster-Hauser Syndrome):
– A congenital abnormality resulting from paramesonephric duct development failure and may be associated with urinary tract abnormality. Clinical presentation includes either amenorrhea or haematocolpos depending on the spectrum of disease

10.3 CLASSIFICATION OF VAGINAL RECONSTRUCTIVE OPTIONS FOR CONGENITAL DEFECTS

Dilatation	– Frank
Split skin graft over a mould	– Abbe–McIndoe procedure
Full thickness skin grafts over stent	
Local flap	– e.g., Labial, fasciocutaneous vulvoperineal, or pudendal thigh
Regional flap	– e.g., Gracilis, vertical, or transverse rectus abdominus myocutaneous flap
Distant flap	– e.g., Pedicled colon

10.4 ANATOMICAL CLASSIFICATION OF ACQUIRED VAGINAL DEFECTS

In Plastic Surgery VI, Ed. Mathes. Trunk and Lower Extremity. Saunders Elsevier; 2006:1296

Type I: Partial
(A) Anterior or lateral wall involvement
(B) Posterior wall involvement

Type II: Circumferential
(A) Upper 2/3 of vagina
(B) Total vaginal resection

Chapter 11
Burns

Epidermal burn:
– *A burn that affects only the epidermis (e.g., Sunburn)*

Superficial burn:
– *A painful partial thickness burn affecting the epidermis and upper dermis, commonly accompanied by blistering*

Deep dermal burn:
– *A partial thickness burn extending deep into the dermis with fixed staining becoming evident 48 h post injury. Potential regeneration due to some skin adnexal structure sparing*

Full thickness burn:
– *A burn extending through the full thickness of the skin and potentially deeper, associated with destruction of all skin adnexae*

11.1 CLASSIFICATION OF BURN DEPTH

| | Partial thickness | | | | Full thickness |
	Superficial	Superficial dermal	Mid dermal	Deep dermal	Dermal
Colour	Red	Pale pink	Dark pink	Red fixed staining	White
Refill	+	+	Slow	–	–
Sensation	+	+	+	–	–
Blisters	–	Small	Large	–	–
Healing	+	+	Usually	–/+	–

Mary O'Brien, *Plastic and Hand Surgery in Clinical Practice*,
DOI: 10.1007/978-1-84800-263-0_11,
© Springer-Verlag London Limited 2009

11.2 CLASSIFICATION OF BURN TYPE

Thermal
Chemical
Electrical
Inhalational
Non-accidental
Friction

11.2.1 Classification of Thermal Burns

Scald
Flame
Flash
Contact

11.2.2 Classification of Chemical Burns

Alkalis (cause a liquefactive necrosis)
Acids (cause a coagulative necrosis)
Organic compounds
Phosphorus

11.2.3 Classification of Electrical Burns

Low voltage <1,000 V
High voltage >1,000 V
Extremely high voltage
  Lightning:
    (a) Direct (fatal)
    (b) Sideflash (hits a tree and then discharges current through the air or ground to an individual)

11.3 CLASSIFICATION OF INHALATIONAL INJURY

Supraglottic
Subglottic
Systemic

Minor burn – <10% TBSA child, <20% adult
Critical site – Face, Hands, Genitalia
Major burn – A burn covering 20% or more of the total body surface area (TBSA)
Extensive burn – >60%
Formal fluid resuscitation burn – 15% adult, 10% child

11.4 PARKLAND FORMULA FOR BURNS RESUSCITATION

4 ml kg^{-1} per percent Total burn surface area
1/2 given in the first 8 h post injury
Remainder given over the subsequent 16 h

PLUS maintenance fluids in children

4 ml kg^{-1} for first 10 kg

+

2 ml kg^{-1} for second 10 kg

+

1 ml kg^{-1} > 20 kg

11.5 URINE OUTPUT INDICATING ADEQUATE FLUID RESUSCITATION

Adult = 0.5–1 ml kg^{-1} h^{-1}

Child = 1.0–1.5 ml kg h^{-1}

11.6 CURRERI FORMULA FOR DAILY CALORIFIC REQUIREMENT IN BURNS PATIENTS

Adult = 25 kcal kg^{-1} + 40 kcal per percent burn

Child = 40–60 kcal kg^{-1}

11.7 CLASSIFICATION OF ZONES OF INJURY (JACKSON'S MODEL 1947) (FIG. 11.1)

Inner zone:
– *Coagulative necrosis resulting in irreversible tissue loss*

Intermediate zone:
– *Stasis, decreased tissue perfusion potentially salvageable with adequate resuscitation*

Outer zone:
– *Hyperaemia*

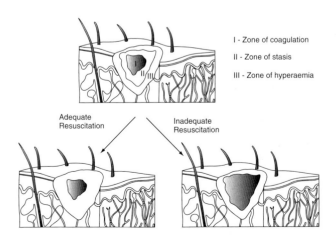

I - Zone of coagulation

II - Zone of stasis

III - Zone of hyperaemia

Adequate Resuscitation

Inadequate Resuscitation

FIGURE11.1. Jackson's zones of burn injury.

11.8 CLASSIFICATION OF PATHOPHYSIOLOGY

Local Effects
1. Release of inflammatory mediators: By capillary wall, white blood cells, and platelets
2. Vessel: Vasodilatation and increased permeability
3. Oedema: Resulting from fluid (protein and trace elements) leak from the circulation into the interstitial space

Systemic Effects (> 20–30%)
CVS – Hypovolaemia, RBC destruction, flame haemorrhages of myocardium
RS – Pulmonary oedema, tracheobronchitis, pneumonia
GI – Loss of protective function, bacterial translocation, curling ulcers therefore prophylaxis
Liver – Peroxidation of hepatocytes
Immunosuppression – Decrease in the mechanical barrier, decrease in non specific and specific (humoral and cellular) immunity
Glucose intolerance – Massive catecholamine release
Clotting deranged – PE/DVT therefore prophylaxis required

11.9.1 CLASSIFICATION OF THE IMMUNE SYSTEM
(a) Mechanical barriers
(b) Non specific immune response
(c) Specific immune response

(a) *Mechanical barriers:*
Skin – Physical barrier
  – Immunological cells (dendritic, langerhans, mast, macrophage, T, PMN)
RS   – Mucociliary staircase
GI   – Mucus, enzymes

(b) *Nonspecific immune response (independent of previous contact):*
Circulating phagocytes – Polymorphonuclear cells (PMN) (neutrophils, basophils, eosinophils)
  – PMN peak at 1 day and 1 week post burn
  – Monocytes (antigen presenting cells associated with MHC I)
Plasma proteins: – Opsonins (enhance phagocytosis)
  – Complement–Classical pathway (Ag-IgM, Ag-IgG activated)
    –Alternate pathway (microbial products activated)

(c) *Specific immune response (previous contact dependent):*
T (thymus) lymphocytes: Cell mediated immunity
Stimulated by Antigen (Ag) presented by Antigen presenting cells (APC)
  T helper cells: release cytokines, attract phagocytes, stimulate B, and
    NK cells
  T suppressor cells: Inhibit T helper cells

B (bone marrow) lymphocytes: Humoral immunity
  Produce Antibody when activated by T helper cells

Natural Killer (NK) cells (Ag MHC I): affect Ig coated viruses/tumour

11.9.2 CLASSIFICATION OF EFFECTS OF BURNS ON THE IMMUNE SYSTEM

Burns affect each arm of the immune system causing immunosuppression at each level:

(a) Mechanical barriers
(b) Non specific immunity
(c) Specific immunity

In addition:
Transfusion induced immunosupression
Steroid induced immunosuppression secondary to endogenous
  glucocorticoid release

"SIRS"
– *Systemic inflammatory response syndrome*
– *Two or more of the following criteria must be present for a diagnosis:*
– *Body temperature >38°C or <36°C*
– *Heart rate >90 beats min^{-1}*
– *Respiratory rate >20 min^{-1} or PaCO$_2$ <32 mmHg*
– *WCC > 12,000 μL^{-1}, <4,000 μL^{-1}, or >10% immature forms*
(Modified accordingly in children)

"MODS"
– *Multiple organ dysfunction syndrome that can be induced by SIRS*

Cytokine
– *A broad group of polypeptides with varied functions within the immune response*

11.10 NATIONAL BURN CARE REVIEW BURN CLASSIFICATION

Complex (require plastic surgical intervention)

Non complex (no immediate specialist intervention required)

11.11 CLASSIFICATION OF BURNS UNIT REFERRAL CRITERIA

(Complex burns)

Significant burn: – Partial thickness burn >10% adult
>5% child
– Full thickness burn >1%

Significant area: Hands, feet, face, perineum, major joints, circumferential

Significant chemical or electrical injury

Significant other: Age extremes, comorbidity, major trauma, non-accidental injury (NAI), inhalational injury

11.12 CLASSIFICATION OF BURN SURFACE AREA ESTIMATION METHODS

(a) Lund and Browder Chart: adult/paediatric
(b) Palm of patient's hand, fingers adducted approximates 1% TBSA
(c) Wallace's "Rule of 9s"

	Head and neck	1 arm	1 leg	Anterior trunk	Posterior trunk	Perineum
Adult	9%	9%	18%	18%	18%	1%
Child	18%	9%	14%	18%	18%	

*Each year >10 year, take 1% off head and add to combined legs

11.13 CLASSIFICATION OF BODY FLUID COMPARTMENTS

Total Body water = Intracellular fluid (2/3) + Extracellular fluid (1/3)

Extracellular fluid = Vascular compartment (1/3) + Interstitial fluid (2/3)

Vascular compartment = Venous component (85%) + Arterial component (15%)

11.14 CLASSIFICATION OF AIMS OF BURN CARE

Summarized from "ABC of Burns" – Blackwell Publishing Ltd 2005 – Hettiaratchy, Papini, Dziewulski

Rescue
Resuscitate
Retrieve
Resurface
Rehabilitate
Reconstruct
Review

11.15 CLASSIFICATION OF TIMING OF BURNS SURGERY

Immediate: Tracheostomy, escharotomy
Early<72 h: Excision & Graft   (a) tangential;
                                          (b) fascial
Intermediate   <1 week   (initial indeterminate depth which fail to heal)
Late   >3 weeks
Delayed reconstruction   (contracture release, scar revision)

11.16 CLASSIFICATION OF BURN DISASTER TRIAGE

Summarized from "ABC of Burns" – Blackwell Publishing Ltd 2005 – Hettiaratchy, Papini, Dziewulski

Group I   – Minor burns in a non critical site
Group II   – Minor burns to a critical site
Group III   – Major burn (20–60%)
Group IV   – Extensive burn (>60%)
Group V   – Minor burn + Inhalational or associated injury

First priority evacuation   III + V
Second priority evacuation   IV
Third priority evacuation   II
First aid/Primary care referral   I

11.17 CLASSIFICATION OF DRESSINGS FOR BURNS

Purposes: – to absorb fluid
          – to decrease pain
          – to act as a barrier to infection

Autograft   – Split skin graft, cultured keratinocytes
Allograft   – Cadaveric skin, fresh or cryopreserved
Xenograft   – Porcine derivative
Synthetic   – Semipermeable membranes, Occlusive,
               Hydrocolloid, Absorptive

Combined   – Allogenic + synthetic membrane (e.g., Transcyte: allogenic cells providing growth factors + scaffold)

Topical   – Bactroban, Polyfax, Flamazine, Flamacerium
agents

11.18.1 CLASSIFICATION OF POST BURN CONTRACTURES OF THE IPJ OF THE HAND

Stern PJ et al. Classification and treatment of post burn IPJ flexion contractures in children. JHS (Am) 1987; 12(3):450–457

I   Deformity correctable by flexing MCPJ
II   Deformity not fully correctable with MCPJ flexion
III   Deformity unaffected by MCPJ position

11.18.2 CLASSIFICATION OF BURN CONTRACTURES OF THE MCPJ OF THE HAND

Graham et al. Classification and treatment of post burn MCPJ extension contractures in children. JHS (Am) 1990; 15(3):450–456

I   Correctable with wrist extension
II   MCPJ flexion <30° with wrist extension
III   Unaffected by wrist position

Fasciotomy:
– *Division of the fascia to release compartment pressure*

Escharotomy:
– *Division of the thick, inelastic burn eschar to aid perfusion of the limbs and ventilation of the chest (Fig. 11.2)*

11.19 CLASSIFICATION OF NATURE OF SUBSTANCES WHICH CAN EXTRAVASATE

Vesicant
Irritant
Neutral

11.20 EXTRAVASATION INJURY CLASSIFICATION OF MECHANISMS OF TISSUE INJURY

(a) Osmotic imbalance: Hypertonic solutions, 10% dextrose, hypertonic total parenteral nutrition (TPN)
(b) Ischaemia induction: Catecholamines, vasopressin
(c) Direct toxicity to cells: Sodium bicarbonate, digoxin, tetracycline

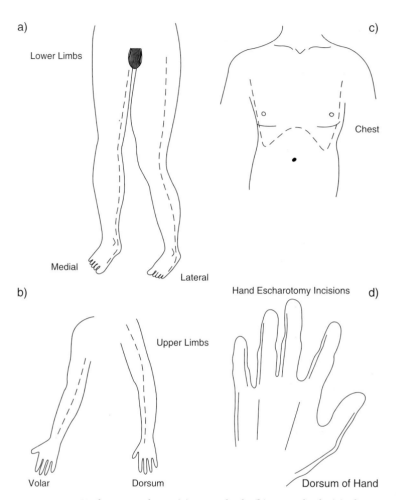

FIGURE 11.2. Escharotomy lines: (**a**) Lower limb, (**b**) Upper limb, (**c**) Chest, and (**d**) Hand.

11.21.1 CLASSIFICATION OF COLD INJURY

Local: – Frostbite
            – Non tissue freezing injury: trench foot, chilblain
Systemic: – Hypothermia

Frostbite:
– A localized cold induced injury usually affecting digits

11.21.2   CLASSIFICATION OF FROSTBITE

First degree   – Whitish plaques, swelling, hyperaemia, causalgia, rare tissue loss
Second degree   – Blistering, erythema, oedema, tissue recovery
Third degree   – Full thickness skin loss
Fourth degree   – Cyanosis, gangrene of deep structures including muscle and bone

11.21.3   CLASSIFICATION OF PHASES OF FROSTBITE

Prefreeze (3–10°)
Freeze–Thaw (–6 to –15°)
Vascular stasis
Late ischaemia

11.22.1   RADIATION INJURY CLASSIFICATION

Acute (industrial accidents)
Subacute (previous therapeutic radiation for malignancy)
Chronic (former therapeutic treatment of benign skin diseases, industrial exposure)

11.22.2   RADIATION WOUND CLASSIFICATION

Dunne-Daly CF. Skin and wound care in radiation oncology. Cancer Nurs 18(2):144–162
Erythema
Dry desquamation
Wet desquamation

Osteitis:
– *Demineralization of bone secondary to osteoblast radiation damage*

Osteoradionecrosis:
– *Infection of bone as a result of irradiation*

Chapter 12
Cosmetic Surgery

Aesthetic unit
– *A functional division of tissue defined by contour lines within which the tissue shares similar characteristics in terms of colour, texture, and quality. Sutures lines should ideally correspond to the boundaries to achieve the best camouflage. If greater than 50% of the aesthetic unit is lost, it may be preferable to replace the whole unit. Some regions may be divided into subunits.*

Body dysmorphic disorder
– *A psychiatric condition whereby a person is preoccupied with a perceived defect in appearance despite having a normal appearance which causes significant distress and may interfere with social, occupational, and interpersonal functioning. Surgery does not cure this condition.*

12.1 THE FACE (FIG. 12.1)

12.1.1 Classification of Facial Changes as a Result of Aging

Histological Changes
Loss of type III collagen
Loss of elastin
Dermo-epidermal junction flattening
Decreased Langerhans cells and melanocytes

Clinical Changes
Quality of skin: thin, wrinkled, skin cancers, pigmentation, excess, loss of elasticity
Brow/eyelid: Ptosis
Wrinkles: crows feet, perioral

Mary O'Brien, *Plastic and Hand Surgery in Clinical Practice*,
DOI: 10.1007/978-1-84800-263-0_12,
© Springer-Verlag London Limited 2009

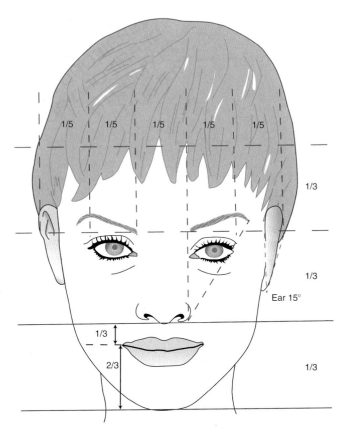

FIGURE 12.1. The ideal facial proportions.

Jowls
Nasolabial fold prominence
Platysmal bands

12.1.2   Classification of Types of Rhytid
Animation creases from insertions of muscles of facial expression

Fine rhytids
Deep rhytids

12.1.3   Fitzpatrick Classification System of Perioral and Periorbital Rhytidosis
Class I   – Fine wrinkles

Class II – Fine-to-moderately deep wrinkles, moderate number of wrinkle lines

Class III – Fine-to-deep wrinkles, numerous wrinkle lines, redundant folds possibly present

Fitzpatrick correlated these three classes with the following scoring system and degree of elastosis:

• Class I (score 1–3) – Mild elastosis
• Class II (score 4–6) – Moderate elastosis
• Class III (score 7–9) – Severe elastosis

Mild elastosis:
– *Fine textural changes with minimal skin lines*

Moderate elastosis:
– *Yellow discoloration of individual papules (papular elastosis)*

Severe elastosis:
– *Marked confluent elastosis with thickened, multipapular yellowed skin*

12.1.4 Glogau Rhytid/Photoaging Classification Scheme
Glogau RG. Aesthetic and anatomic analysis of the aging skin. Semin Cutan Med Surg 1996;15(3):134–138

Group I:
Mild (age 28–35 years) – Little/no wrinkling, no keratoses, no scarring, requires little or no makeup for coverage

Group II:
Moderate (age 35–50 years) – Early wrinkling, sallow complexion with early actinic keratoses, requires little makeup, mild scarring

Group III:
Advanced (age 50–60 years) – Persistent wrinkling at rest, discoloration of the skin with telangiectasias and actinic keratoses, always wear makeup, moderate acne scarring

Group IV:
Severe (age 65–70 years) – Severe wrinkling, photoaging, gravitational and dynamic forces affecting skin, actinic keratoses with or without cancer, wears makeup with poor coverage, severe acne scarring

12.1.5   Facial Aging: A Clinical Classification

Shiffman MA. Simplified Facial Rejuvenation, Chap. 5. Ed Shiffman, Mirrafati, Lam. Springer; 2007:65

Stage	Tear trough depth	Cheek fat loss	Nasolabial fold depth	Jowl prominence
0	None	No loss	None	None
1	Slight: to cheek fat	No loss	Slight	None
2	Mild: into cheek fat	Slight loss medially	Mild	Slight
3	Moderate	Moderate	Moderate	Moderate
4	Severe	Severe	Severe	Severe

12.1.6   Classification of Facial Layers

Skin
Subcutaneous tissue
Superfical musculoaponeurotic system (SMAS)
Fascia/muscle
VII Nerve

Superficial musculoaponeurotic system (SMAS):
(Mitz and Peyronie)
– *A layer of facial fascia continuous with galea, frontalis, temporoparietal fascia (superficial temporal) and platysma. With a couple of exceptions the motor nerves lie beneath and the sensory nerves lie above*

Sub-SMAS plane (deep plane):
– *The plane between the superficial and deep facial fascias which includes the deep attachments of the facial muscles, retaining ligaments of the face, areolar spaces and branches of the facial nerve*

12.1.7   Classification of the Retaining Ligaments of the Face

Derived from Furnas DW. Plast Reconstr Surg 1989;83:11
Osteocutaneous:
– Zygoma
– Anterior mandible

Musculocutaneous:
– Platysma – cutaneous
– Platysma – auricular

McGregor's patch:
- *A fibrous band from periosteum of zygoma to dermis*

Pitanguy's line:
- *Surface marking of the frontal branch of the facial nerve*
- *Runs 0.5 cm below tragus to 1.5 cm above lateral eyebrow*
- *The nerve becomes superficial and lies just beneath the temporoparietal fascia*

Rhytidectomy or facelift:
- *A procedure used to correct the cervico-facial changes that occur with aging*

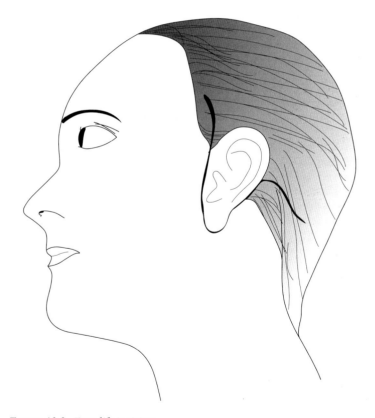

FIGURE 12.2. Face lift incision.

12.1.8 Classification of Facelift Techniques
Skin lifting alone
Skin and SMAS/ platysma
Deep plane: composite flap of skin and SMAS (Hamra PRS 1992)
MACS Lift: minimal access cranial suspension surgery
Midface suspension
Non endoscopic subperiosteal facelift
Endoscopic facelift

Turkey gobbler neck:
– *Divarication of platysma causing unsightly platysmal bands at the medial border*

Witch's Chin deformity:
– *Ptosis of chin skin and subcutaneous tissue.*

12.1.9 Classification of Facelift Complications
Intraoperative
Early
Late

12.1.10 Facelift "SCAREs" Classification
CM O'Brien

Skin- necrosis 1–3% (×12 in smokers), scarring, swelling, seroma, bruising
Changes in pigmentation: haemosiderin deposits
Alopecia, asymmetry
Residual bleeding giving rise to haematoma 3.7%
Excessive tension: dehiscence, infection, ear lobe deformity
Significant nerve injury
– Great auricular nerve (commonest sensory nerve involved)
– Buccal branch of facial nerve (commonest motor nerve involved)
– VII (0.9%)
– (Facial numbness)

12.1.11 Classification of Secondary Face Lifts: Goals
Relift
Remove old scars
Preserve temporal/sideburn hair

12.1.12 Classification of Facial Danger Zones
Zone 1: Great auricular nerve – 6.5 cm below the external auditory canal

Zone 2:   Temporal branch of VII – Pitanguy's line
Zone 3:   Marginal mandibular branch of VII – 1–2 cm below lower border of mandible
Zone 4:   Zygomatic/Buccal branches of VII – anterior to parotid and posterior to zygomaticus major
Zone 5:   Supratrochlear/Supraorbital nerves – superior orbital rim above mid-pupil
Zone 6:   Infraorbital nerve – 1 cm below inferior orbital rim mid-pupil
Zone 7:   Mental nerve – mid-mandible below second premolar

12.2 THE NECK

12.2.1 Classification of Neck Types

Dedo D. A preoperative classification of the neck for cervicofacial rhytidectomy. Laryngoscope 1980;90(11 pt 1):1894–1896

Class I	Well defined submental angle, little submental fat, good skin, and platysma tone
Class II	Early laxity of cervical skin without significant submental fat or loss of platysma tone
Class III	Subcutaneous layer of fat
Class IV	Platysmal abnormality is the predominant change + /– pre- and sub-platysmal fat
Class V	Retrognathia
Class VI	Abnormally low hyoid

12.2.2 The Five Youthful Neck Criteria

Ellenbogen R, Karlin V. Visual criteria for success in restoring the youthful neck. Plas Reconstr Surg 1980;66(6):826–837

1. Acute cervicomental angle (105–120°)
2. Distinct inferior mandible border
3. Subhyoid depression
4. Visible thyroid cartilage
5. Visible anterior border of sternocleidomastoid

12.3 THE BROW

12.3.1 Brow Lift Classification of Approach

Endoscopic

Open
   – Suprabrow excision
   – Bicoronal brow lift

- Frontal hairline brow lift
- Temporal brow lift
- Transblepharoplasty brow lift
- Browpexy

Combined

12.3.2 Ellenbogen Criteria for the Ideal Brow
(Fig. 12.1)

Brow starts: Vertical line through the alar base
Brow ends: Oblique line joining the alar base and lateral canthus
Horizontal plane connects medial and lateral ends
Apex of brow: Vertical line through the lateral limbus
Position of apex of brow: Women – just above the supraorbital rim
         Men – at the level of the supraorbital rim

12.4 BLEPHAROPLASTY
(Also see oculoplastic section in Chapter 5)

Blepharoplasty:
- *A procedure to modify the appearance of the eyelids by removing excess skin and removing or redraping excess fat (Greek derivation: "blepharon" = "eyelid") (Figs. 12.3 and 12.4)*

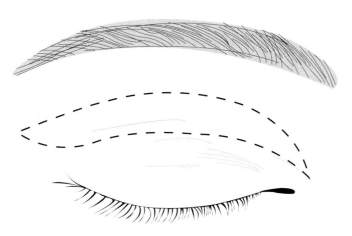

FIGURE 12.3. Upper lid blepharoplasty incision.

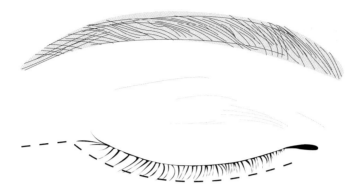

FIGURE 12.4. Lower lid blepharoplasty incision.

Compensated brow ptosis:
- *Compensatory contraction of frontalis when opening the eyelids to counteract the descent of the eyebrow evident upon closure of the eyelids (Blepharoplasty worsens the appearance if compensated brow ptosis is present)*

Snap test:
- *After gentle distraction of the lower lid from the globe, it should snap back into position within a second, if not it indicates lid laxity*

Bells phenomenon:
- *Upward movement of the globe on eye closure*

Canthopexy:
- *A procedure to restore the lower eyelid to its normal position, tone and tilt*

Retrobulbar haemorrhage:
- *Bleeding behind the orbital septum which can lead to pressure on the globe and irreversible blindness. It may result from trauma or rarely as a result of iatrogenic injury during orbital surgery (0.04%)*

Chemosis:
- *Excessive oedema of the conjunctiva*

Tear trough defect:
- *Primarily a bony defect causing the appearance of deep grooves at the junction of the eyelid and cheek skin*

Nasojugal groove:
– *Primarily a muscular deficiency (orbiclaris oculi and levator labii superioris alaque nasi) causing the appearance of deep grooves at the junction of the eyelid and cheek skin*

12.4.1 Classification of Differences Between the Asian and Caucasian Upper Eyelid

Adapted from Park DH, Kim YK. Blepharoplasty Techniques In Asians. In Simplified facial Rejuvenation, Ed. Shiffman, Mirrafati, Lam. Chap. 60, p. 467

Anatomy	Caucasian	Asian
Lid crease (%)	100	50
Origin of medial lid crease	Medial eyelid	Medial canthus
Tarsal height (mm)	9–10.5	6.5–8.0
Septum-levator fusion point	Above tarsus	As low as the pretarsal plane
Preseptal fat pad location	Preseptal	Preseptal, pretarsal

12.5 RHINOPLASTY

1. Nasolabial angle	100–110° (women)
	95–100° (men)
2. Mang's angle	110–120° (formed by the intersection of the nasal root-to-tip and nasal tip-to-chin lines)
3. Glabellar angle	35°

Rhinoplasty:
– *A surgical procedure to alter the appearance of the nose*

Bony vault:
– *Area overlying the nasal bones*

Cartilaginous vault:
– *Area overlying the upper lateral cartilages*

In fracture:
– *Medial movement of nasal bones to correct an open roof deformity*

Infratip lobule:
– *Area from the tip to the start of the columella*

Lobule:
– *Area overlying the alar cartilages*

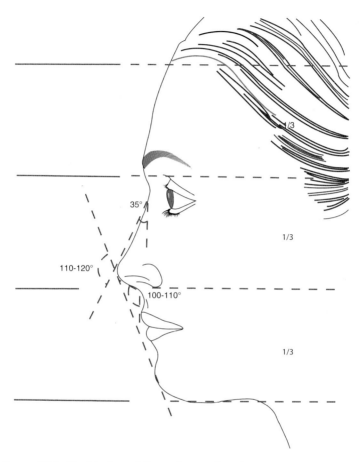

FIGURE 12.5. The ideal nasal dimensions and angles.

Nasal length:
– *Distance between the nasofrontal groove (root of the nose) and nasal tip*

Open roof deformity:
– *The flat, wide appearance of the dorsum after removal of a dorsal hump without in fractures*

Out fracture:
– *A fracture which mobilizes nasal bones prior to in fracture*

Soft triangle:
– *Rim of nose that does not contain cartilage and separates the dome from the nostril border*

Supratip:
– *Area just above the domes of the alar cartilages*

Tip defining points:
– *Most prominent areas of nasal tip: domes (right and left), supratip, columella break point*

Tip projection:
– *Distance from the nasal spine to the nasal tip*

12.5.1   Classification of Nasal Anatomy

Upper third   – Nasal bones
Middle third – Upper lateral cartilages (lie posterior to nasal bones and alar cartilages)
Lower third   – Lower lateral (alar) cartilages

12.5.2   Rhinoplasty: Classification of Technique
Open
Closed

12.5.3   Classification of Rhinoplasty Incisions (Fig. 12.6)
Rim (vestibular border)
Intercartilaginous: between the upper and lower lateral cartilages
Intracartilaginous: splitting of the lateral crura of the lower lateral cartilage
Transfixion: through the membranous septum
Alar base excision

12.5.4   Classification of Osteotomies Performed During Rhinoplasty (Fig. 12.7)
Low to high
Low to low
Double level

Internal nasal valve angle:
– *The angle between the upper lateral cartilages and the septum (10–15°)*

Valve area:
– *Circumference of airway at the level of the internal nasal valve*

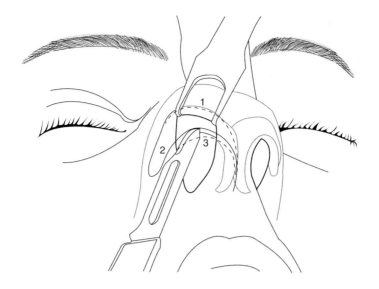

1 Vestibular border incision (Rim incision)

2 Intracartilaginous incision

3 Intercartilaginous incision

FIGURE 12.6. Rhinoplasty incisions. 1 Vestibular border incision (rim incision). 2 Intracartilaginous incision. 3 Intercartilaginous incision.

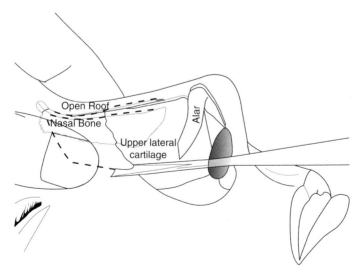

FIGURE 12.7. Nasal bone and cartilage relationships with osteotomy lines indicated.

Spreader grafts:
– *Cartilage grafts between the septum and upper lateral cartilages which increase the internal nasal valve angle improving respiration*

Umbrella graft:
– *A strut of vertically placed cartilage between the medial crura from the nasal spine to the nasal tip on top of which is placed an onlay graft*

Nasal cycle:
– *The normal 3 hourly congestion decongestion cycle*

Cottle sign:
– *Lateral cheek traction opens the nasal valve and improves air entry*

Pinocchio tip:
– *Excessive nasal tip projection*

Parrot beak deformity:
– *Inadequate nasal tip projection in association with a high supratip*

12.5.5 Classification of Suture Technique to Adjust the Nasal Tip
Transdomal
Interdomal
Lateral crural mattress
Intercrural
Columella – septal

12.6 ABDOMINOPLASTY

12.6.1 Abdominoplasty Classification System of Diagnosis and Treatment
Matarasso A. Clin Plast Surg 1989

	I	II	III	IV
Skin laxity	Minimal	Mild	Moderate	Severe
Fat	Variable	Variable	Variable	Variable
Musculofascial system flaccidity	Minimal	Mild lower abdominal	Moderate lower or upper	Significant lower or upper
Treatment	Liposuction	Mini	Modified abdomino-plasty	Standard

12.6.2   Huger Classification of Zones of Arterial Supply to the Abdomen (Fig. 12.8)

Huger WE Jr. The anatomic rationale for abdominal lipectomy. Am Surg 1979;45:612

Zone I   Deep superior and inferior epigastric arteries
Zone II   Superficial epigastric, superficial external pudendal, superficial circumflex iliac systems
Zone III   Segmental perforators: intercostals, subcostal, lumbar arteries

12.6.3   An Aesthetic Classification of the Abdomen Based on the Myoaponeurotic Layer

Nahas FX. Plast Reconstr Surg 2001;108:1787

A. Rectus diastasis secondary to pregnancy
   Treatment: Plication of anterior rectus sheath
B. Rectus diastasis and laxity of the infraumbilical aponeurotic layer
   Treatment: Plication of anterior rectus sheath and L-shaped plication of the external oblique aponeurosis
C. Congenital lateral insertion of the recti muscles
   Treatment: Release and undermining of the recti muscles from the posterior sheath and midline advancement
D. Rectus diastasis and poor waistline
   Treatment: Plication of anterior sheath and advancement of external oblique

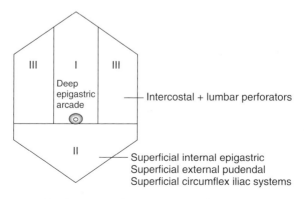

Figure 12.8. Blood supply to the abdominal wall.

12.6.4 Classification of Types of Abdominal Contour Deformity and Treatment

Bozola and Psillakis

Bozola AR, Psillakis JM. Abdominoplasty: a new concept and classification for treatment. Plast Reconstr Surg 1988;82:983

Type 0 Normal contour
Treatment: None
Type 1 Excess fat only
Treatment: Suction assisted lipectomy
Type 2 Infraumbilical skin excess, + /– fat excess, muscle taut
Treatment: Mini-abdominoplasty
Type 3 Infraumbilical skin excess, + /– fat excess, may have infraumbilical musculoaponeurotic layer laxity
Treatment: Mini-abdominoplasty
Type 4 Infra + /– mild supraumbilical skin excess, + /– fat excess may have overall laxity of musculoaponeurotic layer
Treatment: Limited, modified or extended mini-abdominoplasty
Type 5 Infra- and supraumbilical skin excess, + /– fat excess, + /– laxity musculoaponeurotic layer
Treatment: Traditional, Classic abdominoplasty including umbilical translocation

12.6.5 Pitman

Pitman GH. In Grabb and Smith's Plastic Surgery. Eds Aston, Beasley, Thorne. Philadelphia: Lippincott-Raven 1997:676

I Excess fat, taut skin, and muscle
Treatment: Liposuction
II Lax infraumbilical skin, taut muscle, +/– excess fat
Treatment: Resect lower abdominal skin and subcutaneous tissue
III Infraumbilical lax skin and muscle, +/– excess fat
Treatment: Infra-abdominal abdominoplasty + muscle tightening
IV Lax muscle, minimal, or no excess skin, +/– excess fat
Treatment: Complete abdominoplasty without umbilical translocation
V Lax supra- and infraumbilical skin, lax muscle, +/– excess fat
Treatment: Complete abdominoplasty with umbilical translocation
VI Circumferential skin laxity severe (secondary to massive weight loss),+/– residual fat, +/– muscle laxity
Treatment: Circumferential abdominoplasty

12.6.6 Other types of abdominoplasty:

Vertical abdominoplasty
Reverse abdominoplasty

12.7 LIPOSUCTION

Liposuction:
– *Aspiration of subcutaneous fat through small incisions by cannulae of varying diameter attached to a vacuum system*

12.7.1 Classification of Technique
Traditional
Ultrasonic assisted
Power assisted

12.7.2 Classification of Liposuction Technique According to Subcutaneous Infiltration Volumes

Dry   – No infiltrate
Wet   – 200–300 cc infiltrate per treated area
Superwet   – 1 cc infiltrate: 1 cc aspirate
Tumescent   – 2–3 cc infiltrate: 1 cc aspirate

Pre-tunnelling:
– *Creation of channels in the allocated area prior to suction to establish an even plane.*

Cross tunnelling:
– *Creation of channels at an angle to those created by pre-tunnelling*

Fountain effect:
– *The jet of infiltrate emerging from a small incision under pressure once tumescence has been achieved*

Feathering:
– *A technique to eliminate steps between suctioned areas and non treated areas*

12.7.3 Classification of Liposuction Complications
CM O'Brien. "LIPOPROBLEMS"

L   Loss of symmetry
I   Infection
P   Perforation (abdominal/thoracic)
O   Oedema
P   Parasthesiae/dysaesthesiae
R   Reactive discoloration
O   Osmotic fluid shift
B   Bleeding
L   Lignocaine toxicity
E   Ecchymoses
M   Mal contour
S   Seroma

12.8 UPPER EXTREMITY BODY CONTOURING

12.8.1 Classification of Brachial Fat Deposits and Skin Laxity
Vogt P. Body Contouring: Upper Extremity in Plastic Surgery, vol 6. Ed Mathes, Saunders Elsevier; 2006:293

Group 1   Minimal to moderate subcutaneous fat
          Minimal skin laxity
Group 2   Generalized accumulation of subcutaneous fat
          Moderate skin laxity
Group 3   Generalized obesity
          Extensive skin laxity
Group 4   Minimal subcutaneous fat
          Extensive skin laxity

12.9 THE BREAST
(See Chapter 7 for breast augmentation, reduction, mastopexy and nipple reconstruction)

Abbreviations

AJCC	American Joint Committee on Cancer
AFX	Atypical fibroxanthoma
Ag	Antigen
AK	Actinic keratosis
AN	Accessory nerve
APL	Abductor pollicis longus
APC	Antigen presenting cell
APB	Abductor pollicis brevis
BCC	Basal cell carcinoma
BMI	Body mass index
CMN	Congenital melanocytic naevus
DCIS	Ductal carcinoma in situ
DFSP	Dermatofibroma sarcoma protruberans
DIPJ	Distal interphalangeal joint
DVT	Deep venous thrombosis
DXT	Radiotherapy
EAM	External auditory meatus
ERCL	Extensor carpi radialis longus
ECRB	Extensor carpi radialis brevis
EPB	Extensor pollicis brevis
EIP	Extensor indicis proprius
EDC	Extensor digitorum communis
EDM	Extensor digiti minimi
ECU	Extensor carpi ulnaris
FDP	Flexor digitorum profundus
FDS	Flexor digitorum superficialis
FNCLCC	French Federation Nationale des Centres de Lutte Contre Le Cancer
FPB	Flexor pollicis brevis
FPL	Flexor pollicis longus
FTSG	Full thickness skin graft
GI	Gastrointestinal
HPF	High power fields

Ig	Immunoglobulin
IJV	Internal jugular vein
IPJ	Interphalangeal joint
ISSAV	International Society for the Study of Vascular Anomalies
IV	Intravenous
LCIS	Lobular carcinoma in situ
MACS	Minimal access cranial suspension
MCPJ	Metacarpophalangeal joint
MFX	Malignant fibrous histiocytoma
MHC	Major histocompatibility complex
MM	Malignant melanoma
MODS	Multiple organ dysfunction syndrome
MRI	Magnetic resonance imaging
MTPJ	Metatarsophalangeal joint
NAC	Nipple areolar complex
NF	Neurofibromatosis
NICH	Non-involuting congenital haemangioma
NK	Natural killer cells
PA	Postero- anterior
PABA	Para-amino-benzoic-acid
2PD	Two point discrimination
PE	Pulmonary embolus
PIPJ	Proximal interphalangeal joint
PVNS	Polyvillonodular synovitis
RBC	Red blood cell
RS	Respiratory system
RSD	Reflex sympathetic dystrophy
RLD	Radial longitudinal deficiency
RICH	Rapidly involuting congenital haemangioma
SA	Surface area
SCC	Squamous cell carcinoma
SCM	Sternocleidomastoid
SIRS	Systemic inflammatory response syndrome
SLAC	Scapholunate advanced collapse
SMAS	Superficial musculoaponeurotic system
TBSA	Total body surface area
TFL	Tensor fascia lata
TMJ	Temporomandibular joint
TNM	Tumour, node, metastasis
TNMG	Tumour, node, metastasis, grade
TMJ	Temporomandibular joint

UCL	Ulna collateral ligament
V	Volts
VPI	Velopharyngeal incompetence
WHO	World Health Organisation
X-ray	Radiograph

Index

Printed in the United States of America